W9-CAG-029

ALSO BY ALEXANDRA HEMINSLEY

Ex and the City:
You're Nobody 'Til Someone Dumps You

Running Like a Girl

Notes on Learning to Run

ALEXANDRA HEMINSLEY

SCRIBNER

New York London Toronto Sydney New Delhi

Scribner

A Division of Simon & Schuster, Inc.

1230 Avenue of the Americas

New York, NY 10020

First Scribner hardcover edition October 2013

SCRIBNER and design are registered trademarks of The Gale Group, Inc., used under license by Simon & Schuster, Inc., the publisher of this work.

For information about special discounts for bulk purchases, please contact Simon & Schuster Special Sales at 1-866-506-1949 or business@simonandschuster.com.

The Simon & Schuster Speakers Bureau can bring authors to your live event. For more information or to book an event, contact the Simon & Schuster Speakers Bureau at 1-866-248-3049 or visit our website at www.simonspeakers.com.

Manufactured in the United States of America

1   3   5   7   9   10   8   6   4   2

Library of Congress Control Number: 2013018909

ISBN 978-1-4516-9712-4

ISBN 978-1-4516-9717-9 (ebook)

For my father, who taught me to put one foot in front of the other.

*For my brother, who has kept me going more times
than he can imagine.*

And for David, who brought me sunshine.

Contents

Running Like a Girl

It's the most natural thing in the world.

We were born to run.

You just put on your shoes and head out the door, that's the beauty of it.

It's just you, the road and your thoughts.

These are the things that people say about running. These are lies.

Running is awful. It feels unnatural, unnecessary, painful. It can hijack you with breathlessness, cripple you with panic, and overwhelm you with self-consciousness. It isn't a warm fire or a deep sofa or a cup of tea and a smile. It is cold and hard and unforgiving.

It is also the pleasure of being outside on a sunny day, feeling the prickle of the sun on your skin. It is the delight of feeling your body temperature rise despite the crisp winter breeze against your face. It is feeling blood rush around every part of your body and coming home to a welcoming bath and a delicious curry, your skin still glowing an hour later.

And, as I have learned, it is an honor, a privilege, and a gift.

Before I get to the "gift" part, I want to tell you about the hard beginning. When I began, I too was repulsed and intimidated by the beatific smiles and radiant smugness of the determinedly Sporty Types. For years, running seemed a punishment—yet another way we were being told to keep off the pounds, to feel the burn, to pay for that half glass of white wine and square of chocolate. God forbid we might have a body that was less than beach-ready!

It wasn't always this way. I could remember how everything just felt more fun and free when I ran as a child. Now that I was a woman in my thirties, who'd spent several years forgetting supper on a Friday in place of a night out, there didn't seem much to encourage me.

So, this book is the one I didn't have but would have liked to read before I went on my first (disastrous) run. Something for those people who think they can't run, for whatever reason. For the women who think they aren't slim enough to wear running tights or that it's not worth it if they don't want to complete an entire marathon, for the women who think that running around in circles is an idiotic way to spend the best part of an hour. For those women who don't trust yet that it really is a source of immeasurable pleasure, self-belief, and unexpected companionship, rather than a necessary purgatory—that they might, just might, enjoy the confidence, the physical ease, or the mental clarity that running brings.

Because it was in running that I found all that and more.

PART ONE

1

Not Born to Run

Only those who dare to fail greatly can ever achieve greatly.

—Robert F. Kennedy

I don't remember making the decision that I couldn't run; it was simply one of those things that made me *me*, like my love of cheese or my distaste for men in turtlenecks.

My certainty that I couldn't run was absolute, my envy profound of those who could, and my admiration for my flatmate boundless. She would appear at the front door, glowing from one of her regular routes around Regent's Park or Hampstead Heath, and I would welcome her enthusiastically. We'd chat about what she'd seen, while she leaned at the kitchen counter sipping a glass of water and I sat on the sofa with my laptop propped on my knees like a windy baby.

"I wish I could run." There is a certain comfort in saying it aloud. "It looks like so much fun," I'd say, sighing, as she took off her running shoes. I felt a twinge of sadness, knowing that it was too late for me to start. I would reach for the TV remote with resignation.

As I watched my flatmate's running clothes circulating hypnotically in the washing machine, I never questioned the casual lunacy of my conviction that I couldn't run. I remember being six or seven and running being what I could barely wait to do during break time at school. And I remember being thirty, having total confidence that running was utterly beyond me. The change had been cumulative, something that I let happen to me, a state of affairs I succumbed to without question.

Somehow I had forgotten the itch in my legs when I was in school, looking up at the clock, back at the teacher, and out of the window. Soon. Then, the very second the bell rang, we would grab our coats and head outside to play whatever game we could think of, as long as it meant running around. We didn't call it running at that age, because running was how we did everything, mittens trailing from our sleeves and braids whipping at our cheeks. We were just children doing our thing. We ran and we laughed. They were one and the same.

As a ten-year-old, I stood daydreaming at the start of the four-hundred-meter circuit. In the warmth of summer, I watched the sun shine through the pinprick holes in my navy blue shirt, noticing how it browned both my arms and the grass of the track. I would merrily run round it for as long as I could, sometimes straight across the middle if I fancied a change, until we were called back to lessons or until someone else needed the track.

Twenty years later, it was as if I had never run. It didn't occur to me that I could. I wasn't a runner, and that was that. Somehow I had lost sight of the fact that not being a runner and being unable to run were not one and the same.

I wasn't the sporty type. It was as simple as that. I was a curvy girl with little or no competitive spirit. I rarely made a connection between bat and ball during games at school, and I neglected my body almost entirely for three years at university. Perhaps I broke into a run that time I was pushing my friend Clare down Cotham Hill in a shopping cart, and I know I danced on a podium a few times, but those were definitely the sum of my collegiate athletic endeavors.

Then I moved to London and joined the eternal treadmill of private gym membership. Each time I looked round a new venue, I told myself that this would be the one. This would be the gym that would make me fall in love with exercise. They never did. Once the oleaginous buzz of viewing the facilities, being given my workout profile, and trying the steam room for the first time was over, the magic faded and I returned to fleeting, guilty glimpses at my bank statement as I realized each visit was costing me more and more.

Back then I didn't know that the gym was just sticky methadone to the heroin of running outdoors. How could pounding along on the treadmill, going nowhere in front of a wall of relentless rolling news, compare to the freedom of running along the seafront, looking up at a hovering seagull and finding yourselves neck and neck for a moment? Still I continued. Next came the (Madonna-influenced) yoga phase. Relaxing, but only as relaxing as it could ever be to race across the city and part with more money than I'd spend on three weeknight dinners for the sake of ninety minutes bending and sweating in front of myriad freelance Web designers and stressed-out fashion editors. Then came Pilates and even a flirtation with meditation.

Finally, after a summer of heartache followed by almost crippling depression, came the walking phase. After a hectic routine of lying under my coffee table weeping, I had reached a point where I had to get outside and see daylight. I wanted to feel the breath of warm air on my skin; I yearned to feel my blood circulate round my body again, and I needed to do it with a view that was not just that of a ceiling tile or a yogi's tatty three-week-old pedicure. Half-deranged by weeks of erratic sleeping—nights spent enervated and panicky followed by sluggish, heavy-limbed days—I decided in desperation that physically exhausting myself might make the nights seem a little more welcoming. I longed to long for my bed, instead of seeing it as a sleepless battleground. I yearned to yearn to lie down at the end of the day, legs aching from use rather than the anxious jiggling they did under my desk for hours on end.

Thus began my walking phase. One day I up and left the house and didn't return until nearly dusk. I began walking for hours at a time. Hampstead Heath, Regent's Park, Hyde Park. I would leave the house on a Sunday morning and not return for three or four hours. Often I could barely remember the time I had spent away, as if the repetitive quality of my strides had hypnotized me. I would begin full of fire, longing to get away from the dirty streets, the dawdling pedestrians, the local shops whose owners had seen me tearstained and bedraggled during my summer of agony and bad eating. As the parks opened up before me, I would feel my spirits lift. I would romp around the heath, deliberately getting lost in a wooded area I didn't recognize. I would stroll through rose gardens, wondering about the stories behind the blooms' names. A tiny part of me I thought I had lost started to wriggle back to the surface.

I arrived home from my walks exhausted but noticeably lighter of spirit. My head felt as if someone had popped in and run a duster around it. I formed a truce with my bed. I cherished my time off the grid, uncontactable and alone. The coils that had spent endless nights tightening in my mind loosened a little; my imagination wandered toward the positive rather than the self-focused disaster-movie scenarios it had devoted itself to. I remain convinced that those walks in the summer of 2006 saved me. Not just because they restored my ability to sleep but because they delivered me that first germ of physical confidence. If I could walk for four hours, what might happen if I sped up . . . and then sped up even more? My heart had begun to believe that anything was possible. I had even let myself entertain the notion that maybe, just maybe, I was capable of going for a run.

It was this expansive spirit of optimism that inspired my first run to Queen's Park a year later. If my heart could survive the pummeling it had taken, my legs must have more to give. I'd been taking three-hour walks regularly for about a year, so I figured I *might* be ready for a run.

That was it. I was going to run round the block. I had high hopes: the ass of an athlete, the waist of a supermodel, and the speed of a gazelle. I had finally bottomed out, defeated by gyms, bored by sanctimonious yoga teachers, and intimidated by glossy tennis clubs. It was time to end a lifetime spent believing that I existed in a galaxy nowhere near the sport's. I would return powerful and proud, the city reeling at the sight of my grace and speed on the pavements of Kilburn. This is the story of my first run.

My preparations were extensive: First there were two weeks of thinking about it. What would it feel like? Would I fall over? How would I get home if I found it too much? I was filled with positivity and enthusiasm. Then I panicked; then I became exhilarated; then I put it off for a couple more days.

It was a Saturday in August, the month of my sister's wedding. It was sunny but not too hot, perfect running weather. That afternoon I was heading to a party in Norfolk with my family for wedding guests who wouldn't be able to make it to the ceremony, to be held abroad. It was the perfect time to get in shape, I told myself. After all, the big day was coming up in a couple of weeks, and I had bribed myself to take that first run on the grounds that I could really get involved with the party food later. Amid the happy chaos of the family wedding to come, I thought it would be nice to have the promise of an empowering new hobby to return to.

When the morning of The Run came, I woke up and immediately ate three slices of toast with honey, for "energy." Then I spent ninety minutes faffing around on iTunes, trying to compose a playlist of such magnitude that it would propel me round the park, no matter how debilitating I found the experience. Despite my extensive research, I didn't dare to buy anything new. Instead I dug out some old tracksuit bottoms, last worn when I'd had adult mumps and watched two *Sopranos* box sets in a single weekend. I rifled through my drawers until I found a bra that covered as much of me as possible. I found some old running shoes in the back of my cupboard beneath some festive reindeer antlers.

There was little else I could do to procrastinate. The laundry was done, the ironing was pancake-flat, the bookshelves dusted. Every possible worst-case scenario had been replayed in my head a million times, and it was clearly never going to rain. I had run out of excuses. I tied back my hair, grabbed a bottle of water, put my keys in the pocket of my tracksuit bottoms, and stood at the front door. This was it. I was going for a run.

I opened the front door and walked down the three steps

to the pavement. What was I supposed to do next? Perhaps some stretching? I held on to a lamppost and pulled my foot up behind me, trying to stretch the front of my thigh. I did the same thing with the other leg and looked around anxiously. My heart was beating too fast already. What if onlookers could tell it was my first run? Would they be able to see that I was doing it wrong?

Running. It was just running. I set off down the road, trying to look to the Saturday passersby as if this were something as normal to me as taking the bins out. But that road was a long road. It was the grouting between the urban delights of Kilburn High Road and the chic coffee shops of Queen's Park. As I headed toward the park, the houses became progressively more glamorous and well groomed. I, however, did not.

I was halfway down the road when I had to stop. There was an awful juddering as the whole world moved up and down on account of my lumbering limbs: thud, thud, thud as my feet hit the ground, sending shock waves through both my body and the pavement. Within seconds, my face had turned puce with intense heat and my chest was heaving. I could see the crossroads, but to my ragged humiliation, I could not make it that far. I was not just out of breath; I was having to swallow down panic to keep myself moving at all.

I walked for the length of the next song on my playlist. The indignity of admitting I could no longer run seemed slightly less than that of the physical wreck I would become if I continued. Eventually, I made it to the park and tried to run for the length of the next song. I could not manage that, so I ended up walking past the field of children playing football at the center of the park. Each of them darted around effortlessly, continually in motion, while every part of my body seized up.

The wobble of my thighs, the quake of my arse, the ridiculous jiggle of my boobs seemed to mock me as the Saturday dads stared in horror from the playground. Every time my feet struck the tarmac, I was convinced my ankle would twist, and every time I looked down to check, I was confronted with the unwieldy expanse of my thigh. My physical self was entirely disconnected from everything my intellectual or emotional self was trying to tell it. *Calm down, putting in the effort is the main thing* was met with *Yeah right, because putting yourself in this much pain is a great idea.*

As I reached the far end of the park and turned to head back, the pounding of my heart and then the slow fire in my lungs convinced me of one immovable fact: I would never make it home.

After several more starts and stops and the total avoidance of eye contact with every person I passed, I got home. It took a good fifteen minutes before my breathing and heart rate returned to normal, and almost an hour before my face stopped radiating heat—and the red glow of a thumb recently caught under a hammer. I stood, slumped at the kitchen sink, gulping water, and remembered the sight of my onetime flatmate, composed as she enjoyed an invigorating post-run glass of water. I was far from channeling her look. But I had done it. I'd been for the megarun, and therefore the spoils of war would be mine. I'd earned them, after all.

Consequently, I rewarded myself handsomely with a phenomenal amount of food and drink at the party that night, blithely telling everyone that I'd been for a huge run that morning.

"It's been a training day for me!" I said brightly to a passing godparent I'd never met as I scooped a second helping of lasagna onto my plate.

"Okay, great," said the relative, nonplussed at my enthusiasm to share details of my sporting endeavor. I was not, after all, a woman who at that point exuded any athletic prowess over the dinner table.

When I woke up the next morning, I felt as if I had been run over by a truck. A big truck with huge grooved tires. This wasn't the pleasing ache of the day spent well on the sports field that I dimly remembered from my youth. No, this was an altogether sharper pain. It felt as if my body were stinging, almost acidic. My limbs were heavy, and muscles I never could have pointed to twenty-four hours earlier were suddenly making themselves known. Oh, this was an unacceptable way to make oneself feel. I must have overtrained. Later, I looked up how far I had run: one mile. My disappointment could not have been keener.

It was another three months before I tried to run again.

When I returned home that Saturday, I felt broken in body and spirit. My lungs and legs were wracked with pain, and my mind had inflicted a thousand tiny blows. Was this what running was going to feel like now? Would every run mean confronting this heinous shame, pain, and rage? Why did people do it? Why did I want to do it? What part of myself was I hoping to access? Slimness, physical achievement, something else? Chastisements rained down upon doubts as I sat, wretched, in the bath. After that disastrous first attempt, these thoughts wedged themselves at the back of my mind for months, like a pen behind an old radiator, always just out of reach.

My sister's wedding came and went in an ecstatic flash. My reaction to the multiple photographs of me, however, was less joyful. Instead of the confident curves I'd always seen myself as having, I realized that part of the juddering agony of that first run was due to the fact that I had put on weight. Running would help with the weight, but the weight did not help with running.

I began to understand what other women meant when they talked about feeling trapped in their own bodies; the magazines I would sniff at in railway stations and doctors' waiting rooms were full of them. I used to think I would never become one—until I found myself watching runners with increasing longing, wondering what their secret was, how they knew what to do, what got them going. Yet running still seemed an impossibility.

Everyone has limitations, and I had reached mine. I was sure of this, though it made me sad. I would see other runners, catch snippets of their conversation as I waited to pay for a coffee, be drawn to their image on magazines or on TV. Increasingly, I was attuned to them in the world around me. Surely, if I stayed alert, I would discover what the secret was that they all knew and I didn't. As I paced the house looking for my lost glasses, I would lift magazines and search websites, hunting for the golden nugget of advice or inspiration to reassure me that a runner lurked in me after all. Because without it, there was no way I could face that Saturday-morning experience again. As the summer ended and the leaves began to fall, I would walk home grudgingly from the tube station, overtaken by the occasional runner, who served only to make my heart heavier. I resolved to try and forget about running altogether. The secret escaped me.

I did my best until a few weeks later, when my siblings and I were staying with our parents for a weekend. My brother casually mentioned that he was going to apply for a place in the London Marathon.

"Wow!" I gasped. "How amazing to be able to do that! I was so surprised when I went to cheer on a friend. It's such an emotional event."

"You should do it too, then," said my father. His voice didn't flicker. He didn't look up from the cup of coffee he was making. His hands remained steady at the task. All very well, coming from a man who'd run several marathons when we were children, but this was me we were talking about.

"Don't be ridiculous!" I exclaimed. "I can't run."

"You *don't* run," he corrected me. "But you're more than able." There was no shadow of doubt in his voice. Hearing it from someone else made me realize: There was nothing stopping me from running but me.

And that was that. The seed was planted.

The next morning I announced that I was not to be broken. August's dismal performance was an anomaly to be forgotten. Indeed, I would run again. I started making a kerfuffle on a scale that suggested I was planning to run home from South Wiltshire to North London. I commanded my father's computer for hours, Googling "small run northwest London," "how to know if you can do 5K," "supplies needed for 5K run," and various permutations of the same.

I downloaded maps, I discussed nutrition and running style with my brother, and I chatted about shoes and bras with my sister. Somewhat exasperated, my father explained that I had two working legs, no medical problems, and a lot of long walks under my belt. He reminded me that it would be about half an hour before adding, "If you get tired, you just walk. You know you can do that."

It was afternoon before I returned to London. By the time I got to the Regent's Park tube station, night had fallen. I hugged the darkness to me, relieved that no one would be able to see the fear on my face. I crossed into the park, made sure no one was around, and set off.

At first it was exactly like the last time: the burning, the panting, the panic. This time there were two key differences: I was not in my neighborhood, so there was little chance of seeing anyone I knew; and I was running a loop, so I *had* to get back to where I had started. After about twelve minutes, a miracle: It got easier. My heart rate, while still high, started to even out. Instead of feeling like a never-ending heaven-bound roller coaster that would only ever go up, I steadied. The two beats of my feet started to match the two beats of my breathing—in and out. I was doing it. Yes, my legs were hurting. Yes, I was scared that I would never make it all the way around the park. But yes! I was running.

By the time I got home from my second run, I was awash with a heady cocktail of endorphins and undiluted smugness. I did some ostentatious stretching with my lights on and curtains open, took a bath (curtains closed), and ate a bowl of pasta approximately the same size as my sister's wedding cake.

It was as if I were experiencing a reverse hangover. The wondrous, magical, heady phase of being drunk lasts for such little time—an hour, perhaps three at best, before it melts into discomfort, delirium, or just plain boredom. Yet the hangover can last a day or two. Finally, I could see with startling clarity that the time I had spent experiencing pain on a run was outweighed by the amount of time that I felt good about it. I was aglow. I was invincible. I was thinking I might be able to do it again.

One of the few concrete pieces of advice my father had given me the weekend before was to keep a running diary so that I could remind myself how I felt after different runs. When I look at that first entry, it says this:

18th October 2007
5K round Regent's Park
5:45–6:20 P.M.

So exhausted after 12 mins. but then it seemed okay. Felt so much easier than expected. Might go again!

The next day I e-mailed my brother. I was going to run; I was going to need a goal to keep me on course. Bumbling around the park indefinitely would not hold my attention, and I wasn't going to see my brother embark on a marathon without me. After all, this might be my only chance for a training partner.

"Hey, do you have that application form for the London Marathon?"

I pressed send.

2

Learning to Run

Anybody can be a runner. We were meant to move.
We were meant to run. It's the easiest sport.

—Bill Rodgers

The idea of me running the London Marathon was of no interest to some and hilarious to others, whose reaction to news of my new hobby was: "You're doing what?" or "Yeah, good luck with that!" or the odd "Ha ha ha, we'll believe it when we see it." The spectrum of reactions created in me determination and terror in equal measures.

Then there was the e-mail from my friend Vanessa, who worked for the charity Sense. Sense is a charity that does amazing work with families of deaf-blind children. Vanessa had been part of the team for years. I had seen photographs of events, I had met her colleagues in the pub, I had heard about families she'd worked with. I knew from her direct experience what a difference fund-raising for them would make, and shifting that focus from me to a charity only cemented my determination to see the plan through.

So it was Vanessa whom I contacted to see if my brother and I could be a part of their charity team. To our amazement, after filling in forms with our fund-raising ideas and committing to do the training properly and raise eighteen hundred dollars each, we were given places on the team. Despite all of this, an e-mail arrived from Vanessa the next day, delicately reminding me that what I had just committed to doing was "quite hard-core."

I had been bold enough to assume that people's tones might change once I had a confirmed place to run. And yes, most *were* encouraging—no one wanted me to fail. But there was an unmistakable sharp intake of breath after I told them my news. A nervous giggle. One too many *Seriously?*s. They tried to be polite, but the responses did little to quell my increasing suspicion that I had taken on something insane, something undo-able, something that remained indisputably not me.

Each time I told someone about the project, I found myself needing a little extra steeliness to protect myself from that uncaught, impulsive mixture of mirth and disbelief. *Why the hilarity?* I found myself wondering time and again. *It's just running, surely there's a cap on how funny that can be.*

Every time I gritted my teeth, bent on doing things properly despite the sniggers, I was seized by fear and acute self-awareness. As a child, I was unself-conscious. My earliest memories of sport were of standing in sunny fields playing softball, waiting patiently for a ball to come my way, or leaping effortlessly around a netball court.

My clumsiness began in my adolescent years. When I was twelve or thirteen and my body started to change, I felt utterly alien from it, as if I'd been deposited in another being's skin. I grew so fast that I spent the better part of a summer crying with pain. On a wretched holiday, I sat on a sandy beach, watching my brother and sister play, as the ratcheting agony of the growing pains in my knees occupied every inch of my mind and body.

At first my family members were sympathetic when I would leave a room and hit a table or a door handle with my hip. Until it started to happen several times a day. Just passing the salt across the dinner table involved knocking over a full water glass with my new boobs, or swiping at a jar of ketchup with my suddenly long arms. I felt like a novice forklift driver, trying to control mechanisms I was inadequately trained to operate.

Sport became torture. The other girls in my class seemed to grow stronger and slimmer as I became more curvy and unwieldy. My body, once a source of such fun, was now more of a straitjacket. When I wasn't fretting about how it looked, I was worrying about what shape it might be next.

I did have a fail-safe weapon in my arsenal: humor. Too proud to let anyone know I cared and too young to worry about lack of fitness, I goofed around during sports. I became the class clown on the sports field. Take a funny pratfall, and no one will mind if you lose the team a goal, I realized. Or mess around enough during tennis lessons, then the girls who can really play won't pick you anymore.

These were easy lessons to learn, and soon I turned those years of loathing into fun. Here began my tacit acceptance that sport was not for me. I was one of the funny girls, the clever girls. I didn't have time for earnest sorts and their sweaty enthusiasm. Sport had slipped, sandlike, from between my fingers.

Now in my thirties, I realized I was paying the price for twenty years of playing the clown. For every pratfall I had taken to prevent anyone taking me seriously on a sports field, there was a giggling e-mail from a friend or colleague, complete with wiseass query about how many vases I might have knocked over stretching, or whether my place for the London 2012 Olympics was confirmed. I might have decided I wanted to be taken seriously, but no one else seemed to be on board with that plan. Despite these reactions, there remained a dusty, barely used corner of my mind where I knew I wanted to prove to everyone what I could do. I wanted to be treated like a grown-up, to be believed when I said I had set myself a goal. I wanted to be respected, not just liked. With a marathon, I saw my window of opportunity. It was just going to take a *lot* of running.

The acceptance of my marathon application meant there was no turning back. I was committed to running regularly, despite having little or no idea what I was doing. Pushing aside the practicalities, I focused on the marathon as a goal and used it as a motivator. I had cheered on friends in the past and been moved by the sight of so many humans trying their very best to do something. I ignored the memories of men running by with chafed-to-bleeding nipples, and feeling quite faint from the heat of a particularly hot April's day despite being a spectator, standing entirely still. I would cross the finish line proud, I was sure of it.

It was this tiny, gritty speck of determination that kept me going in those early days. My running diary from the autumn of 2007 is filled with entries that say little more than "Well, it started fine but then I got INCREDIBLY TIRED" or "My legs felt like actual lead until the last ten minutes—why bother?" or the charmingly pragmatic "This run was so awful I don't want to record it."

Perhaps I kept the diary because I wouldn't believe I had done the runs otherwise. My father had recommended it as a way to remind myself what I thought I was capable of and seeing it change.

This was before the advent of smartphones and running apps, so I would map my runs online before leaving the house, having scribbled up my arm the order of the street names I needed to follow. I cared less about getting lost than I did about being seen. There were too many jokes. Phoebe from *Friends*, *Forrest Gump*, and *The Littlest Hobo*. They all haunted me as I scuttled through side streets, residential roads, and the shadiest corners of local parks, convinced that all passersby could spot my rookie status from five hundred meters. Avoiding eye contact at pedestrian crossings, I kept my cap on and my eyes down, lest I see one of *those women* summing me up.

It wasn't that I wanted to *be* one of them—the lean, toned women who resembled those in the sportswear catalogs, their golden limbs glinting and their ponytails swishing—I just didn't want to exercise anywhere near them. I would lose concentration when one ran toward me. I would feel the edges of my running shoes clip the edge of the pavement if one shimmered through the park. I would feel my stride become irregular if I heard one approaching from behind. After a while, I began to realize that *no one was watching*. Everyone was ultimately more interested in themselves, their children, or their mobile phones. As I discovered when I started trying to smile at approaching runners, quite a few were so tired that they weren't focusing on anything at all.

It amazes me now that I kept leaving the house for those crucial early expeditions, particularly as any potential rewards seemed so far away. I tried whatever I could to maintain momentum, even though I had no real idea what I was doing. I was too proud to ask for advice, lest I give away how much I cared. Google became my friend, and I found myself talking online to novice runners on the other side of the country about where specifically their ankles were hurting. I walked and ran, I ran in tiny bursts, I ran after dark when the sidewalks were emptier. I downloaded podcast after podcast so I could pretend I was doing research for work while I stomped along in my own sweaty world. I kept going, I kept going, I kept going.

After two or three weeks of doggedly jogging around north-west London, I stood on my dusty bathroom scale. "Oh, I never weigh myself! You can't quantify what I am in pounds or ounces!" I remembered telling my mother and sister with a flourish the previous Christmas.

I looked down at my feet and saw that I had shed a few pounds. Later that week, during an idle moment queuing in my local supermarket, I picked up a two-pound bag of potatoes from my shopping cart and let its heft sag in my hands. I had already lost the equivalent of one of those. I imagined the bag strapped round my hips and pictured myself trying to run like that. No wonder half an hour of running felt easier; there was simply less *me* to carry around. Running began to slide, slowly but surely, from a torment to a joy.

What I didn't know on those early runs—the ones where even my face seemed to hurt when I got home—was that I wasn't lily-livered or weak-willed. Nor was I biomechanically unable to run. I was, in fact, "going lactic." As we run, oxygen is constantly being flushed through our bodies, but when there is a shortage of oxygen, the body goes into an anaerobic state and creates lactic acid. The buildup can remain in our muscles, creating that charming run-over-by-a-truck sensation. It stings, it burns, it makes you hurt from your fingernails to the roots of your hair. I had no idea what pace I should be going when I started out. My goal was simply not to die before the end. As a result, I burned myself out by going anaerobic before properly warming up. For weeks I suspected I was able to run for only ten minutes. I would belt out the distance as fast as I could, determined not to walk. When I got home, I'd collapse and descend into existential torment.

I want to weep when I think of the number of women who head round the block only to return twelve minutes later, broken and tearful. I don't doubt that when these women meet me and hear that I have run five marathons, they want to weep for me as well. I suspect that they believe all runs, forever, are as crippling as those first few; that's certainly what I thought. They are not. If only someone had told me sooner.

Except someone had told me sooner: my father. Though it had been his calm acceptance that I could run a marathon that gave me the courage to apply for a place, I had become reluctant to let him in on the mission. That may have been on account of his great eagerness to help. The minute places were secured for me and my brother, our dad offered his thoughts about training plans, anaerobic exercise, and the importance of stretching parts of the body that I'd never heard of. Little of this meant anything to me. While my brother seemed to absorb the basics of the science at a precocious speed, I was stuck on the emotional basics of running.

With the particular charm of an independent-minded, first-born daughter, I sharply informed my father that this was *my* project, it was about reaching *my* goals, and it would be dealt with *my* way. The response was a gentle smile that I half remembered from my tiny hand pushing his away as I tried unsuccessfully to tie my first pair of sneakers for myself. That, and a quiet "Okay then."

A week or so later, when I blithely described to my father how dreadful I was finding my runs, he gently suggested that, as the distance of 26.2 miles was my goal, I should be trying to steadily increase how far I could run rather than attempting a series of bizarre sprints around my neighborhood. Perhaps he had a point. However, I was reluctant to let him take over my project. I looked instead at the training plans in the marathon book I had bought and barely opened. I started to understand the importance of working at a pace rather than running for as long as I could without collapsing. (At this point, there might have been a murmur of thanks in my father's direction, but it was very faint.)

I started to plan the route for each run as a loop, so I had no choice but to complete it, even if I had to walk. Encouraged by an increasing number of e-mails and texts from my dad, and the training plan from the team at Sense, I worked out that I should be running shorter distances during the week and long (or endurance) runs on weekends, increasing the distance incrementally. Long runs required the most planning and levied the strongest emotional hold over me. In an attempt to work out my pace and avoid getting lost, I'd recite street names the whole way round, remembering which turn corresponded with which mile. These days the apps you can download to your phone or iPod are excellent. They monitor your warm-ups and cooldowns and keep tabs on your heart rate, calmly talking you through the interchange of walking and running, making sure your heart rate is elevated and has a chance to recover, rather than blasting on all cylinders and running out of steam. Six years ago I was trying to figure it out on my own, like a crazed Victorian inventor discovering electricity—with running shoes on.

As the weeks wore on, my ramshackle training plans seemed to work, though I was plagued by fears almost every time I reached the end of my road. It was no longer the fear of ridicule; rather, it was that I would be facing down a longer distance than I ever had in my life. I'd stand at the front door, carefully curling my headphone wire round the back of my neck, internally muttering that this would be the one to finish me off: Seven miles was definitely the killer, and I must be crazy to contemplate nine and a half.

Ever more elaborate disaster scenarios played themselves out as I approached the limit of what I had run the week before. There were the standard trips, sprains, and breaks. (Mine were always embellished with some sort of humiliating clothing rip, exposing me to the residents of a particularly chichi street.) There were the Lost Run dreads: the fear that I would somehow circumnavigate London with no sense of space or time, apparently unable to recognize my surroundings or get home. Then there were the vomiting and diarrhea terrors. What would happen if I were sick in the street? Or if I needed the loo? What if I ate something untoward and had to pay the lavatorial consequences five miles from home? Would anyone understand? Greatest of all was my inexplicable yet all-consuming fear of dehydration or hitting the Wall.

It is entirely impossible to read anything about running that does not hammer home the importance of hydration, and there is no literature on marathons that fails to discuss the so-called Wall, the notorious point when your body has expended all of its stored energy and has yet to convert any of the food or drink you've taken in. The idea of losing control haunted me. Scenes flickered across my mind of my body shutting down as I blacked out from dehydration and exhaustion. I pictured my face turning putty-gray as I lay—probably on one of London's most historic streets—foaming at the mouth, publicly flailing, alone. People would laugh and point, sneering, "That's what happens if you don't train properly" or "She probably didn't have enough water" or, most shaming of all, "She clearly took on more than she could manage with *that* distance." There was no doubt in my mind that it would happen one day.

It has never happened.

Things that *have* happened to me: I have tripped on a sidewalk and fallen; I have ripped my running tights; I have realized halfway through a run that the elastic in my running tights has gone; I have gotten lost and had to retrace my steps a little; I have become very hot; I have become very thirsty; I have become very tired.

To date, neither my bowels nor my bladder have inflicted a roadside betrayal. As a child I often longed to be stung by a wasp, just so I could know for sure how much it hurt—so I could stop bloody worrying about how much it might hurt to be stung by a wasp. I felt the same about needing the loo while running. It was a momentous day when, about three months into my training, I was on a cold uphill run through Kilburn cemetery when it hit me that I was going to need a bathroom long before I was home. Beloved Kilburn cemetery, which I found so uplifting, so inspiring, such a wonderful place to run. I simply could not shit there. But for at least ten minutes I thought I was going to.

My brain was whizzing. I ran a finger around the elastic of my jogging bottoms. Could I get them down with one hand, or would I have to put my iPod in my mouth and my keys in my hair? I would have to move fast. I couldn't do it. By now every time I hit the path, a judder went straight up my legs and rattled my sphincter. I could not last much longer. Was it a bigger risk to walk and thus delay my arrival somewhere more suitable, or to run and keep the judders going? I went for a sort of tiptoe run, as if silent footfalls would con my ass into containing itself that little bit longer. I turned and crossed the top of Kilburn High Road, realizing it was only five or ten minutes to home, and all downhill. Not even that convinced me I was going to make it. The potential horror of knowing that I had crouched beside a noble Victorian artisan's grave was replaced with the grim vision of running down Kilburn High Road smelling like a sewer.

Time sped up. I ceased to think of anything but the most basic survival. I spotted a pub on my side of the road and knew it was my only hope. There was no time left for me to fret about the fact that I had been scared of that pub and everyone I'd ever seen going in or coming out of it for three years. As I made those final few strides toward its saloon-style doors, I pushed the sights I'd seen at those doors as far from my mind as possible. There was no time to dwell on the fight I had witnessed midafternoon on St. Patrick's Day between two men barely able to stand, or the stream of doorman-sized fellows I'd seen squaring up to one another after a particularly important rugby match had finished being screened inside. As for the toothless old guys whom I'd spotted on the rare sunny day when the doors were left open, they'd have to go too. My choice was simple: Pull myself together and be prepared to encounter some of Kilburn's shadiest faces, or soil myself.

I was at the saloon doors. I made a sort of martial-arts gesture, chopping across the wire of my headphones so that the earbuds pinged out as I entered the pub. Still moving at quite a canter, I kept my eyes trained on the back of the venue and whipped straight past the barman, who was standing alone polishing a pint glass with a dishcloth.

"I need to use your bathroom, I will explain in a minute!" I yelled as I whizzed by, iPod wires windmilling behind me. Within seconds I was on the loo, stomach gurgling with relief. The heat of the building mixed with the crippling shame of my dramatic entrance meant that I was puce, even by my already ruddy standards. I took a deep breath and tried to run a hand through my hair, sticky with sweat. Mercifully, as I exited, the barman was deep in conversation with a customer and I was able to give an airy wave and a cheery "Thank you *so* much, you're incredibly kind!" before bolting for the door.

As I headed home, running faster than I ever had, a thought struck me: The ability to run was actually useful. Not just for raising money for charity, or for losing enough weight to fit into a dress you thought you never would, but for getting somewhere fast. My legs seemed to be gobbling up the pavement as I headed out of the pub I had been so scared of for so long. That day I could have outrun anyone in the building. I was high on the realization for hours afterward, as well as feeling huge relief at having made it to the bathroom at all.

With the clarity afforded by hindsight, I can see that my father had told me pretty much all of what I eventually worked out for myself in my new running existence, up to and including bathroom anxieties. I didn't listen. I would see him open his mouth and hear words coming out of it, but before any of those words reached me, I would launch into my own "Just because you've done this doesn't mean that I can't do it; I'm in my thirties now, you're not the boss of me, I will find out this information for myself because I am a strong, powerful, and independent woman and times have changed since this was YOUR thing" speech.

As I discovered when I did turn back to him for help, the feeling of swallowed pride is not dissimilar to that of lactic acid.

3

Wicking Fabric and How to Style It Out

Don't bother just to be better than your contemporaries or predecessors. Try to be better than yourself.

—William Faulkner

*T*he great thing about running is that you don't need a whole load of fancy equipment. You just pop on some running shoes, and off you go!

But which running shoes?

For a few months, I ran in a pair of shoes I had bought to celebrate one of my ill-fated gym-membership phases several years earlier. They had been a purchase made entirely based on style rather than on practicality—they'd merely matched some workout gear I was fond of in my early twenties. I'd wear them with the gear and carry a small bottle of water for most of a Saturday morning before deciding time was pressing and I should start to focus on plans for that night's party. It's fair to say that these shoes were experiencing a rude awakening.

Toward the beginning of my training, my father exhorted me to get a pair of shoes that were slightly too big. This seemed like nonsense. Instead of thanking him for his advice, I did my best to brush him off, to end the conversation. What could he know about running shoes? Had he forgotten that only a couple of weekends ago, he was telling us how he ran his first marathon in a pair of Dunlop Green Flash? My siblings and I had chuckled, half awestruck, half-appalled, as he recounted the story of his first marathon, from the can of Coke he was given by the organizers as an energy drink, to the minutes he spent lying on the side of the road for a break, to the fact that he wore through his Dunlops until the sole was flapping off.

My father hadn't had the typical baby-boomer experiences of music festivals or traveling the world. He'd joined the army and had children at a very young age; I was present in my stroller at his graduation from the Defence Academy at Shrivenham. His travel had been done with us, his family, in the form of many military postings abroad and the places he could visit from them.

It seemed that he had found his Woodstock in running. Like a hippie dad telling his kids not to get high on the wrong sort of weed, he had found an audience in me and my brother, and he was keen to share tips and wisdom from the early days on the scene. My brother, a more confident athlete, was happy to listen and take away from the chats what interested him, but I was flailing between what I needed to know, what was relevant in my dad's experience, and what my own stubbornness was prepared to let me listen to.

While I was starting to appreciate my dad's somewhat Zen approach to running, there was one area where I decided his advice had been rendered almost obsolete in the twenty-five years since his marathon prime: gear. What was a hobby for my dad was now a market. When my fund-raising pack arrived from Sense, I realized what an industry running had become.

For every piece of information I sought—whether it was about training plans, socks, or moisturizer—there was someone trying to sell me something. I had no idea whom to trust or where to turn for real objective advice. I had no idea what half of the products were for, or that there were solutions to niggles I'd discovered. It took me two weeks of wearing new running tights to discover the perfect credit-card-sized pocket discreetly folded into the waistband. Time and again I realized I had no idea what was worth buying. Even the language used in reviews seemed utterly alien.

What is a new hobby if not a shopping opportunity? Before long, I had tops that looked good but ruched up above my waist the minute I started to move. I had trousers with pockets designed for a use I had yet to figure out, and I had a rain jacket with a tiny hole above my collarbone that mystified me—until I made the happy discovery that it was meant to keep my head phone wires from flapping in the wind. But in the meantime, I was still trying to run with my fists full of coins, keys, and a subway card, as well as my iPod.

As the weeks peeled away, I became increasingly obsessed with getting the right gear. Partly because I was wearing the clothes so often that it seemed insane not to like what I was wearing, but also because a hunter's instinct had kicked in. As I waded across my flat, now a forest of drying Lycra, every radiator decorated with socks like an athletic Christmas tree, I continued to wonder whether I'd chosen the right products. I wanted to be more nonchalant about this. I wanted to be the sports-shop equivalent of the cool girl who walks into a bar and challenges the boys to a game of pool. I wanted to be able to hold my own during a chat with the lads. (There were no lads for me to have gear chats with, but still.) Unfortunately, I was far from cool.

Just as I was desperate to find gear that would make my training easier, I also wanted to look good without—crucially— looking like I was trying too hard. There was that goofy school- girl inside me, whispering, "Don't try too hard. If you dress like a dork, no one will expect anything of you. Just stick to black."

At least for now there was one thing I didn't need to address: running shoes. Or so I thought.

Apart from the ceaseless quest for the perfect outfit, things were looking good. My confidence was on the up. I could run for over an hour without praying for death, and I had learned some survival basics. I was not going to dehydrate like a novice raver halfway around Regent's Park. I was not going to let the money in my pocket fly off across the river. I was not going to get lost between the Heath and my house. As Christmas approached, I dared to let myself believe that I might—*might*—be able to see this plan through.

Until I did my first ten-mile run. I had been simultaneously looking forward to and dreading it. While I was excited about conquering double digits, there seemed innumerable reasons to pull up the duvet and stay home. It was already well into the festive party season, and I was feeling a little delicate. I was half- way through a crime novel I was spellbound by. I had fresh cof- fee in, and someone had recently given me a box of peppermint creams that I hadn't finished. However, the ten-mile milestone was ludicrously enormous and had to be passed.

The statistics rattled around in my head, becoming more mind-boggling with every spin. I was about to run ten miles for the first time in my life. Ten! And after only a few months of training. I absolutely knew that if I didn't get it done this weekend, it wouldn't happen until after Christmas, and that by then it would be almost impossible.

All it says in my running diary about this run is: "Very cold. Very windy. Very horrible." It was the sort of Sunday that was made for lying in bed with someone you really, really fancy, feeding each other high-carbohydrate foods and talking about novels that, for that day, you truly believe are meant for you and you alone. Instead, I was wearing a selection of ugly, garish clothes, including my old tatty sneakers and a pair of fleece gloves I'd borrowed from my sister.

It had to be done. It had to be done. It had to be done.

I set off down Maida Vale with the list of relevant street names scribbled on the back of my hand. My skin chafed with cold every time I peeled back the glove to check that I was going the right way. I crossed the canal, headed through Kensington, and turned in to Hyde Park. It was bleak, gray, almost deserted. A few old men were resentfully walking the small dogs of wives who had remained indoors. A lonely-looking father pushed a sleeping baby round and round the pond as I ran in the opposite direction. Another runner, a young guy, flashed past me and vanished into the distance down a path near the bandstand.

My ears were raw with cold. I took the glove off one hand and tried to fit my fist in my mouth to warm it up. I wiped my bare palm across my upper lip and realized that my sweat had frozen into little salt crystals across my face. I was miserable. I headed out of the park by Queensway, and the road started to incline slightly. Every time my foot hit the pavement, it hurt more and more. It felt as if the pads of my feet were entirely flat, leaving me running on near bone. I began to wince with almost every stride. My toes were the only part of my body that felt hot; now they were almost radiating. I'd never experienced this level of pain, apart from slamming my thumb in the car door as a wriggling child. The practicalities of my efforts no longer stacked up. If I felt so much pain in ten miles, what would twenty-six feel like? I was barely running, just trudging along, muttering "Keep going keep going keep going" to myself, as condensation poured from my mouth.

I was two and a half miles from home—nearly there. Six months before, I couldn't run two and a half miles. Being nearly there was an enormous feat in itself. This thought alone propelled me onward, despite my throbbing feet.

Eventually, tearfully, I made it home. My hand, clawlike with cold, took over a minute to unlock the front door. I made myself a bowl of pasta, had a long bath, finished my book, and only then looked at my feet. They seemed normal, if a little rosy. Two of my toes were very tender, like a bruised steak. It wasn't until I swung my feet out of bed the next morning that I spotted two of my toenails were dark blue.

My toes looked as if they had been hit with a hammer, cartoon-style. They had not been hit by a hammer; they had simply been for a long run. I had not run on any different or unusual road surfaces. In fact, I had made an effort to avoid running on the cement, which I'd heard was bad news. Over the following days and weeks, I watched with fascination as fresh new nails grew on two of my toes: Each one began beneath the existing nail, from just a couple of millimeters to a full-sized toenail, slowly pushing off the dead nail. It was mesmerizing. After a couple of days I felt no pain at all, merely intrigue. Would the old nail fall off before the new nail was fully grown? Would I have twelve toenails now? Would the new nail grow back in time to paint my nails for spring? These questions consumed me. Until it was happening to my own feet, I had always assumed that the dreaded process of losing a toenail from running would involve the nail coming clean off one day, in a spurt of blood and gore. But no, nothing ever hurt as much as the day of the ten-mile run. I continued through the party season, giving my open-toed shoes a wide berth. A few months later, my new toenails were good to go.

A brief scan of the Internet suggested that I needed some fresh shoes after all. I discovered what had really happened: I had given myself two blood blisters from running in shoes too small. When you run for longer than about twenty minutes, your feet start to swell up, just like they do after a night of fearless dancing in heels you swore fitted brilliantly when you bought them. If you're adding that pressure to the constant slap of foot on unforgiving concrete for a couple of hours, you do in fact replicate the same injury as slamming your thumb in the car door. The thud of toes pressing between trainer toecap and road had been a mighty slam for me on that ten-mile run. It was time to face the music.

Dashing out to buy the right pair of running shoes seemed about as possible as popping down to Denmark Street to buy myself the right Fender Stratocaster. I was clueless. All I knew was "Not too much pink and not too many reflecty bits, like a cheerleader in the eighties, please." Though vanity and my quest for respect stopped me from wanting shoes that looked "fashion," I had no idea whether I could pull off anything more professional-looking. But I knew where to go. To the experts! So, enthusiastic little ponytail swishing in the rain, I headed to the London Marathon store in London's Covent Garden.

On the fascia outside the store is a large digital clock that counts down the days, hours, and minutes to the next London Marathon. I had worked in Covent Garden for years and given the clock an occasional glance at most. I used to laugh on occasion at the earnest expressions of the men within (for they were always men) as I swerved past on the way to a post-work cocktail. Now I needed that store. I needed it urgently.

It seemed best to push aside my quibbles about the store looking very much like one in which a woman had never set foot, and I told myself now that I was a runner, I would be accepted by the staff as one of them. I expected a warm welcome, a kindly listening ear for my queries, perhaps to be addressed in the manner of a colleague or, at the very least, a like-minded spirit.

As I tripped down the street, my nerve started to fade. The numbers flickered above the doorway, counting down. The numbers of days until the marathon seemed very few indeed. Anxieties I thought I'd left behind crept back in. By the time I crossed the store's threshold, my jaunty gait was all but gone. The glass doors clanged shut behind me, and two men looked up and stared as if I were the newest cowboy in a particularly choosy saloon. These weren't the kindhearted fellow runners I had been hoping to encounter.

I nodded to them with strained casualness. "Hi," I mumbled. I edged over to the clothing, circling my target gently. I picked up a couple of tops, ran their curious slithery fabric between my fingers, replaced them on the rack. I held a pair of running bottoms up to my waist, then hurriedly hung them back up. They would no more fit me than an elephant. The younger of the two men approached me. He was wearing serious sportswear and a cap. His tracksuit looked as if it had seen a track rather than just a sofa and some pizza boxes. His gait was confident; he knew his stuff. And he seemed to know I didn't.

"Can I help you?" he asked, as if unconvinced that he could.

"Yes, actually, I am looking for a pair of running shoes." A dramatic pause. I stared him in the eye. "Because I am running the London Marathon."

I awaited the gasps of admiration. Or at least a grunt of camaraderie. Nothing. Not even a shrug. It dawned on me that he probably dealt with chumps like me every day.

"If you're going to buy running shoes, you'll need to be measured, and we only do that by appointment, and we don't have an appointment for a few weeks."

"It's okay, I know what size I am."

"It really doesn't work like that." He had not maintained eye contact. I was starting to sweat; I felt a telltale line start to appear down the back of my T-shirt. I pulled at it frantically.

"How *does* it work? I know my shoe size, and I need some shoes." This young chap wasn't going to get the better of me. I had money to spend, and I was determined to spend it.

"Well, you'll need to run on our @£$@£ machine, and then we'll need to look at your gait and analyze the data, and then @!$£^, and in case of pronation pfftng."

Meaningless words were flapping around me. I had no idea what he was saying. Stress was buzzing in my ears like a wasp in a jam jar. "I'm sorry, could you explain that again?"

He repeated himself. He did not explain. Ennui dripped from his every word. He gestured to a scanlike running machine in the corner of the store. This wasn't going to be like when I was taken to the shoe store as a child to get the new school year's T-bar shoes. My T-shirt was now sticking to my rib cage, front and back.

"Well," I said with a heavy intake of breath as I tried to summon my very best Holly Golightly face, "thank you for your time."

"You need to make an appointment."

I had no intention of making an appointment here; I was scared witless, intimidated by his talk of footfall and pronation and exhausted by trying to maintain the pretense that I belonged here.

"Yes, thank you, I will call in once I have spoken to my assistant." I have never had an assistant. I just wanted to go home and put on my slippers. This shop needed to not have me in it anymore. But I stayed for a further two minutes, occasionally lifting and examining a pair of display shoes. I tilted my head in a manner that I assumed indicated great pensiveness, as if I knew what I wanted yet had decided not to get it today. That was very much the impression I told myself I was giving.

Perhaps it wasn't as long as two minutes, but the burning shame rendered my cheeks a deep shade of crimson, and I left the store sweating and confused. Why had I felt so humiliated? How had one sneering shop assistant managed to make me feel like such an imbecile for wanting something perfectly commonplace and fundamentally sensible?

Over time, my wretchedness turned to rage. How dare they patronize me? They were there to sell me a product. They had the knowledge that I clearly needed to access; why were they obstructing my path? For weeks, months even, I went on thinking that buying running shoes was a rite of passage, an almost mystical experience, an earned privilege.

That is bullshit.

Politeness is politeness in whatever context it occurs, and it is an essential business practice. I can say with confidence that the bloke in the store was either having a very bad day or was just a dick. There is no excuse for being rude to timorous first-time runners, for making them feel stupid for not knowing the correct terminology when they have approached you for help. It takes a lot of courage to go on those first few runs, and either scamming or demeaning them when they are vulnerable and in need of support is unforgivable.

But I'd been cowed for the moment, so I didn't buy any shoes and went bra shopping instead.

Finding a decent sports bra is as important as getting a decent pair of running shoes. Mercifully, I worked this out sooner rather than later, thus avoiding a nipple-related equivalent to the fate that befell my dearly departed toenails. Wearing the right bra is essential no matter how big or small they are. If, like me, you are a cartoonish size 30FF, you are going to need some hard-core scaffolding.

The good news is that there *are* some products that can all but stop your boobs in their tracks for hours at a time. These products don't have to be bizarre combinations of sports and "normal" bras worn over each other, as I have heard some women prefer for running. I have lost count of the number of times women have breezily told me that they can't run because of their boobs. For all that I love my boobs, they are willful and curious, always seeking a new direction to bounce around in and ever keen to seek attention on the Brighton seafront where I can least deal with the stares. But even the most unruly breasts can be contained. Yes, they can.

During my illustrious years of halfhearted yoga and listless gym attendance, I don't remember what sports bras I wore, but they were as primitive as they were attention-grabbing. In short, they were insufficient. It was only the relaunch of the Shock Absorber in 2000 that persuaded me I could take on any sort of long-term exercise without taking someone's eye out.

Though I can't presume to speak for women with smaller bra sizes than mine, the problems of running with a fabulous yet unsupported rack are manifold. Even when you lose a little bit of weight, your boobs will still be there, and they'll start to look even more *there*. Which can be a problem. Boobs are magnificent; you can rest cups of tea on them, feed your children with them, and bring joy to mankind with them, so it really is more than a small shame when something so practical starts to feel like a burden. No one should be burdened by her knockers.

It is distressing to be exhausted toward the end of a run, experiencing the doubt that you'll ever make it, only to find a grotty old man staring at your boobs as if he's found some long-forgotten treasure under a sofa cushion. It is humiliating to see teenage boys or children snigger and whisper as you pass, when you know you'd command their respect in any other environment. It is cringeworthy to see a girlfriend catch her boyfriend copping a quick look when you have done nothing to provoke it. And it is frankly disconcerting to be running along the seafront toward two handsome men, holding hands, clearly a couple, both staring at your untamed breasts.

The worst thing about running with big boobs in the wrong bra is the feeling that you're doing actual harm. That feeling turns out not to be misguided. I have had more than one physical therapist tell me that most women do more harm to their body while running in the wrong bra than in the wrong shoes. Terrifyingly, when you run, breasts don't just do the cartoonish up-and-down bounce; they make a figure-eight movement.

While you might think that stopping the simple bounce is enough, sports bras are working even harder than that. The real risk of running around unsupported is to your Cooper's ligaments. Named in the 1840s after anatomist Astley Cooper, these ligaments are what protect the structural integrity of the breast. Breast tissue is heavier than the fat surrounding it, so these suspensory ligaments keep the tissue from sagging or becoming a megaboob. It's best to look after them, as it is understood that once they are gone, they are gone.

Then there's the chafing. A bra that is even slightly ill fitting will be unbearable after five miles, and that's not accounting for added abrasives like rain and sweat. A small eyelet or hook coming undone can feel like someone jabbing a knitting needle in your back, and the slightest unraveling at a seam can be a disaster in sagginess.

A quarter of women wear a sports bra that doesn't fit, and those are the ones wearing a sports bra at all. The reason most women give for not being properly measured for bra size is that they find it embarrassing. Having suffered my first humiliation at the shoe store, I was more than a little trepidatious, but boobwise, I experienced excellent customer service. I went to a shop where the staff members go to something called the Boob Academy, which is an academy I can get on board with. The prospect of going to a specialist sports outfitter and trying on a random series of boxed sports bras while men stood three meters away, discussing wicking fabric, was out of the question. Given that you can almost definitely burn up to three hundred calories just in the act of getting into a sports bra, the endeavor of purchasing one needs to be undertaken in a calm, restful environment.

My first run in the Shock Absorber bra was life-changing. It felt like home. I am in no way exaggerating when I say that it changed not just my approach to running but my entire outlook on what I might be capable of. I was snugly bound in a manner not dissimilar to that of Judy Garland in her little blue and white pinafore in *The Wizard of Oz*. My boobs were pressed to my chest, but unlike with the bra I had been wearing for running, they were not pushed up under my chin. And I was free from that repulsive splayed effect that can only be described as "what you might see if I were lying on a glass table and you were lying beneath it."

I felt as if my legs and feet were finally free to create momentum that might push me forward, rather than engineer propulsion to encourage my boobs into ever more exciting formations. Similarly, my arms were available to move my body in the right direction, rather than being on standby as emergency dignity shields. It was liberation like I had never known.

My devotion to the bra is such that when my first one reached the end of its life—after what I estimated was over 250 miles of running—I took it apart to see how it was made. It was comprised of seventy-two parts. Seventy-two! Hooks, eyelets, slings within slings, and huge padded arm straps. Each bra is a work of art, available for around forty-five dollars, and I still mourn the demise of my original one. A sentimental favorite. Shock Absorber bras are the result of considerable research begun in 1994 and updated recently, and I remain slightly obsessed with them, as they represent such a huge milestone in the development of my running.

My gleeful bra-based liberty was not without its woes. There is one element to sports bra wearing that I had to work out for myself: Sweat is really, really itchy. Imagine absentmindedly rubbing the deliciously crunchy granules of an expensive salt scrub over freshly shaved sensitive skin. That's the level of pain that can be inflicted on a pair of boobs unprepared for running. If you're running for over an hour, either on a sunny day or under some nice warm layers, you will create little gullies of sweat in all sorts of unexpected crevices. The sweat will dry in salty patterns. And the tiny granules of salt will rub.

For the first few runs I did prior to true bra enlightenment, I thought that the stinging was some sort of allergy to the fabric my bras were made of. I would collapse at home, panting, and hurl the bra from me as fast as I could, shrieking about how free I felt. For two or three days, I would have a tiny ring of pinprick-sized blisters around my rib cage and over my shoulders, where the bra had been working the hardest. After a while five or six small scars appeared.

Over time I have learned that the double whammy of a well-fitting bra with a nice dollop of Vaseline underneath is the answer. (More sophisticated and discerning runners swear by Body Glide, but Vaseline served me well and I recommend it especially for beginners as it's a product most people have on hand.) As for those scars, I used to be terribly self-conscious about them, but now I am of the opinion that there is enough else in the area to distract, and if that doesn't work, I choose not to care. They're battle wounds; they're part of me. They are a minuscule price to pay for the thousands of dollars that I have raised to help those in actual pain.

My boobs were now part of the team, working with me and not against me. In truth, they weren't going to get out much unless I tackled the gruesome problem of new running shoes.

My horrendous experience at the Marathon Store might have put me off indefinitely had it not been for a training day organized by London Marathon that my brother dragged me to just a few weeks later. There was a series of lectures on pacing, training, injury, and nutrition in a university hall. It was the first time I had seen other potential runners. I was terrified at the prospect of viewing them all in an enclosed space, lithe and confident.

The reality could not have been further from the truth. I arrived very late, freezing cold from spending half an hour trying to park my Vespa in the January wind, and finally found my brother. We sat through the morning of interesting lectures, but my mind inevitably wandered, and I found myself studying the faces—and bodies—around me, trying to work out what sort of a runner everyone was. I was shocked and relieved by the staggering diversity of bodies. Not everyone looked as I'd imagined real runners would look.

At lunchtime it was revealed, to my immense joy, that there was a roomful of running-shoe fitters. The marathon sponsor was Adidas, so the brand options were limited, but to my joy, the staff members were very different from those at the London Marathon store. I was asked to take off my running shoes and run across a sensor. Then I returned to where the assistant was standing, and he showed me on a large screen the way my feet fell. There, in flaring red, were the exact spots that had hurt so much on that dastardly ten-mile run. He gently pointed out to me that for the last three months, I had been running in shoes that were almost threadbare. No wonder it felt as if the pads of my feet were worn flat. They were. As for my toes, in shoes that were half a size too small, they didn't stand a chance. I was advised that for long-distance running, I should buy shoes half a size too big to allow for the foot to expand. I sat down and waited for my brother to come back from his fitting. He reap-

peared twenty minutes later with a grin. He'd been told he was
making all the same mistakes I was.

At the end of the training day, we left with running shoes
that fitted properly for the purpose we were intending to use
them. Not everyone needs to get measured immediately or
to make as great an emotional odyssey out of the experience
as I did. But if you do end up running more than every now
and again, you need to buy sensibly. The Adidas shoes that I
bought were perfect; my feet felt like Mariah Carey's might after
a professional rubdown. And I love them for what I achieved
in them. Today they are in a state of terminal filth, and I'd be
repulsed to wear them again. They sit in my parents' garage,
driving my mother mad, but I know they're there, and I like
knowing that they are there.

Once the clouds of my shoe stress had parted, it seemed obvious that the entire university hall was filled with people as desperate as I was to discover that they were not alone—that they
weren't the slowest or the fattest or the ones with the least information. We were all in it together. I was awash with relief. When
I expressed this to my brother, he agreed heartily before adding,
"But it's not as if we don't know anyone who has run a marathon."
I frowned, confused, before I remembered: our dad. I thought of
him that first time in his Green Flash. He had worn through the
soles by the end of the race, but I didn't recall ever having heard
him complain about it. Indeed, despite the story being extraordinary, I believed that we were the only people he had shared it
with. His approach to running was so simple, so self-sufficient.
While I was hanging on to support wherever I could find it—
from the team at Sense, the Internet, a magazine I found on the
train—my dad seemed to have a firm grasp on the key fact: Only
you can run a marathon. No one else can do it for you.

* * *

Still, I remained loyal to the idea that the perfect running outfit could do a couple of extra miles for me. With the twin pillars of running shoes and a bra in place I moved on to socks. Getting a decent pair is an absolute must.

How complicated can socks get? I went for a few runs in the rain in regular socks and found out firsthand. These raw weekend runs taught me just how much a sock can chafe once it has been drenched; they persuaded me to invest in some double-lined sports socks. Effectively two socks attached to each other in some sort of never-ending megasock, they remove the friction from your feet, ensuring that any necessary rubbing goes on between the two layers of fabric rather than fabric against skin. A revelation! And don't get me started on compression socks, something I thought was a fad until I ran a marathon and discovered the sweet, sweet relief that they bring. They feel like leg hugs, comforting and warming in equal measure, as if you have your feet up even when you don't. I have been known to wear them to shows.

Once socks had given me the confidence to swagger around a sports shop asking for what I needed, I was free to experiment with buying all sorts of other products. The more I shopped, the more comfortable I became around the weird and wonderful world of sportswear design while testing the boundaries of what worked for me. I was intrigued by how I might juggle everything I needed for the longer runs. For months I diligently left the house with a sixteen-ounce bottle of water only to return home under an hour later with it unopened. You don't always need it. Unless it's a very hot day, you will be fine for about an hour as long as you've had a good couple of glasses before you leave the house.

For those longer runs, there is a variety of options, from the ergonomically pleasing sixteen-ounce bottles with a hand-shaped grip, to the high-tech backpack-style devices that carry a couple of quarts, feeding a straw into your mouth when you need it. A good friend told me years later that when she undertook her longer runs, she left small water bottles at the foot of trees she would pass, drinking them as she went. For me, the simplest solution was to warn my friends that I'd be stopping at their homes for water along my runs. Otherwise, I'd pop into cafés where the staff knew my face.

In those early days when I obsessed over the disasters that could befall me on anything longer than a 5K run (being hit by a car, passing out from exhaustion, becoming delirious with dehydration, crapping myself in the gutter, et cetera), I continued to leave the house with keys, cash for a cab, iPod, and water. I'd get home with a sodden fiver and the imprint of my front-door key on my palm where it had been pressed up against the water bottle. These days I take keys and iPhone in my hand, having lost patience with those armband holders long ago. They always seemed to slip down to my wrist within three miles.

I'm glad I made those early forays into the world of running gear, though I've changed my mind about a lot of it since. One thing I have remained steadfast on is never wearing shorts to run. I'm not sure I will ever be able to face my raw thighs looming toward me every time I take a step. They are chunky at the best of times, and when I've been running for longer than about ten minutes, they tend to turn a color that even a diplomat would have to describe as corned beef. Add to that the uncomfortable sensation that "loose" legs make as they hit the ground, and it's all too much jiggling for me. I stick to capri-length leggings for most of the year and have a couple of pairs of long running tights for winter to prevent red raw ankles. I have a pair of heavenly thermal-lined running tights for winter, much to the disapproval of my brother, who is insane enough to run in shorts all year round.

The only problem to be solved once committed to running in leggings is that of underwear. Big, sporty, cesarean-height, a thong like a cheese wire—the list of available options is almost infinite. I tried large sporty-branded types first, but I was left dispirited by the enormous dent that the seam—even from seamless ones—left beneath my running tights. The thong lasted no longer than two runs: It is impossible to get farther than three miles looking and feeling as uncomfortable as only having a piece of brightly colored cotton wedged between your butt cheeks while you run up a hill can make you. The solution I found is simple but effective: I no longer wear panties for running. It's just another unnecessary layer beneath a far superior layer of wicking fabric.

I finally worked out what wicking fabric is. Rather than being what my mother describes as "that disgusting slithery stuff," it is in fact a highly technical fabric that moves moisture away from the body and toward the upper surface so as to dry quickly.

When I first envisioned myself running, I saw myself as Jodie Foster's Clarice Starling in the opening scenes of *The Silence of the Lambs*. So strong, so focused, so proud. She is utterly confident, completely single-minded about her training run across a terrifying assault course. At one point she runs past a tree with the sign HURT AGONY PAIN LOVE IT stapled to it. She doesn't care what she looks like; she has shit to do, and she is going to get it done. And yet . . . she is wearing a phenomenally impractical outfit. She is in a heavy cotton sweatshirt and tracksuit bottoms and is drenched in sweat. The top is sticking to both her chest and back and looks painfully heavy. She is summoned by a colleague and heads inside past a roomful of people dressed in khaki, faffing around with guns, and then gets into an elevator. All in the heavy, damp cotton. That wet fabric must have gotten incredibly cold the minute she stopped running, and it bothers me whenever I think of the poor woman in that meeting. For years the scene was my running inspiration, yet now I am unable to watch the first hour of the film without worrying about whether Clarice is shivering from the horrors of Hannibal Lecter or because she caught a dreadful chill.

Mercifully, fabrics these days have eradicated such issues. While modern running tops might seem oddly slithery to the touch, they feel like an entirely different prospect once they're clinging to your chest, protecting you from sweat. Same goes for light-reflective patches on sleeves, necklines, and along the edges of calves and thighs. They are not there, as I initially suspected, as ridiculous splashes of flashing bravado but to potentially save your life on a dark winter's evening.

In the early days, my instinct was to buy and wear clothes as baggy as possible in an attempt to conceal my amateur blubber. I quickly realized how futile that is. Running clothes are not tight because retailers want you to be exposed. They are just easier to run in, and you're less likely to get your headphone cables tangled in loose fabric. And, well, smaller clothes are less fabric to carry around with you or have rubbing against your shoulders, hips, or rib cage as you battle through the rain on a stormy day. I am in no way suggesting than an early-Britney crop top is ideal for every runner, but we don't need to skulk around in a T-shirt that our husband or brother would no longer deign to sleep in.

When I first started shopping for running gear, I would frequently stand in a changing room, heart racing and hair damp with sweat, muttering darkly about why all these clothes were "clearly designed for skinny women who are already fit." I would wail about it incessantly to anyone who would listen, but the fact is indisputable: There is something out there for everyone. I have hunted for skorts with friends who have recently had babies, discovered tiny zips and pockets that are designed to be the same size as a subway card or a spare tampon.

No one designed running clothes to make you feel bad. Why should we look like crap because we're trying hard? I don't believe we should. Increasingly, sports brands are realizing that for as long as exercise is presented to us as a vile must-do to be robotically fitted in between earning a living and maintaining relationships, we're going to resist it. Next time you waver at the threshold of a sports shop, don't think of it as buying clothes to exercise in; approach it as getting some gear to make your body as happy and joyful as possible. It doesn't matter if nothing matches or it gets ripped or splattered in mud—just enjoy wearing it, and let your body have some fun. You should not have to choose between being a runner and being yourself.

4

We Are Family

It is a wise father that knows his own child.

—William Shakespeare

several months after I started running, I realized it was time to start listening to my dad.

I have always loved and respected my father, though he's not one of life's big chatters. Apart from family and his military career, I knew little about what made him tick. Far from a cold man, he is simply very self-contained—and used to a home filled with a wife and two daughters who could marathon at chatting itself, leaving him and his son for dust.

My mother is effortlessly glamorous, as well as somewhat exotic. Raised in the West Indies, she came to London as a teenager and became a dancer. She is rarely not wearing lipstick. She is the kind of woman who painted her nails a fresh specific color before each of our births. And she made staying slim seem effortless. I never saw her sweat. In hindsight, I can see she was on the move from the moment I was awake until long after I fell asleep in a constant flurry of child care and housework. On an emotional level, she can be a bit "turned up to 11."

In adolescence, my body changed, and I became curvy, like my mom. I relished it. She was the epitome of grown-up elegance, and I would stare up from my seat on the carpet behind her, mesmerized by her putting on makeup. Or I would perch on the edge of the bed, enthralled, as I watched her choosing clothes before going out. I aped these little rituals when I grew older, painstakingly applying the cheapest and most basic moisturizer that she finally relented to buy me. I would swoosh the unnecessary cold cream over my face, sweeping it across the area where I hoped my cheekbones would grow, desperately hoping that this would launch me into full adulthood.

Meanwhile, my father seemed to become more distant, or at least different. When I was a child, he had been everything I could ask for in a father. He was endless fun in the garden, constantly inventing games, never tiring of lifting and throwing us from bike to swing and back as we shrieked and gallivanted. He always had time, and he always had energy. Once I had outgrown prancing around, what we had in common decreased at speed. I wanted to chat about lacy bras and makeup, not tanks and foreign policy. As I discovered boys and developed a taste for their associated dramas, it didn't seem terribly cool that my dad was a polite, charming, and kind man.

As I headed into my twenties, our relationship seemed fixed. I loved my father, but I didn't really know how to communicate with him. I accepted this status as permanent and gave it little further thought. Until I bought a copy of *Runner's World*.

As part of my exploration into the world of running, I had timorously bought my first copy of the magazine at a busy train station. I instantly set about reading it from cover to cover. A couple of mornings later, I swung my legs out of bed, pushed myself up in a fog of sleepy limbs, and skidded a foot across the room on the magazine's glossy cover. I looked behind me at the creased pages and headed to the kitchen. As I closed my eyes, waiting groggily for the kettle to boil, I saw a clear image of the permanent heap of running magazines that my father kept on the floor at his bedside. I remembered trying not to skid on them as I clambered up into my parents' bed on Sunday mornings. I remembered one time slipping on them and sending a cup of coffee flying across the carpet. I remembered my mother trying to tidy them up, time and time again. "Why must they be here in the bedroom?" "They are so ugly!" "I keep skidding on them!"

I smiled slowly to myself. I felt a tiny morsel of what it was like to be my father.

A few weeks later, I tried to leave my flat, only to trip over a heap of running shoes by the front door, drying on a sheet of newspaper after a particularly rainy run. An image of my mother doing the same thing at home flashed across my mind. Suddenly I could remember every crease of those mid-eighties New Balance shoes. They were the sort of running shoes that forty-something men who have nonspecific jobs in digital content agencies now wear to the office. Back then, however, they were my father's most prized possession.

Not long after that, I discovered the joy of a long, silent bath after another of my longer-than-I'd-ever-run training sessions. As I closed my eyes and rested my head on the back of the tub, I recalled my sister and me hopping outside of the family bathroom, rattling the locked door handle, desperate for our father to come out and play in the garden. Our mother ushered us downstairs with a stern "You know how tired he is after a marathon." He ran marathons and then came home to a family of three loud and rambunctious children? Of course he did, I realized. He did it several times.

My childhood was reedited. My father was in shorts for breakfast most mornings not because he dressed like us but because he had just returned from a run. We played the best games in our garden because our dad was the fittest, the strongest. The downstairs bathroom was not only where our mum kept a spare bottle of perfume but also where his increasing collection of marathon medals hung.

The next time I called home, I stopped him when he did his usual "I'll get your mother for you." I said, "Hang on, I want to ask you something. How many marathons did you do in the end?" *It must have been five or six all in all,* I thought.

"Nineteen," came the reply.

"Nineteen?!"

"Yes."

"I don't remember you doing half of them."

"Well, I did nineteen official ones, but sometimes I used to do runs that long as well."

"Oh my God. How, HOW?"

Soon we were having one of the longest chats we'd had in months, possibly years. All at once we had a way of communicating, and over the weeks that followed, it became a secret language. He would call me with news of compression socks he had discovered, or supplements, or training tips. We would chat about how my latest runs were going, and I would ask him for advice and motivation. He would cut things out of the paper and send them to me, or save books he had found for the next time I visited home. It didn't matter that sometimes I had no real news about my fitness; it became something we always chatted about anyway, our common ground. It was now "our thing."

Increasingly, he was the only person who kept me going on some of those long runs, the thought of how he had gotten up every morning for years and done it with so little fuss that the most my mother had to complain about was slipping on a magazine. All that time I had thought that we were so different, my father and I. Yet the first time I saw a photograph of myself running, I could pinpoint the exact mid-eighties snapshot of my father that it reminded me of. These legs were his. It was his lungs that were powering me up hills. And it was his quiet acceptance that "yes, running can be hard but is worth it" that was helping me get through the most desperate moments of my training.

My mother maintained a sort of detached bemusement, which in turn amused me. I would come home for the weekend and spend an hour poring over maps at the kitchen table, trying to work out a great training run. She would stare across the room with the same benign lack of interest that she had displayed twenty years earlier when a new pair of New Balance running shoes arrived. My dad ordered them from the States, and they took weeks to arrive via the military post to whichever army base we were stationed at. The day he brought them home was always exciting. New running shoes! Back then I thought that the excitement on his face was entirely unmatched by the gray practicality within. I smiled and remembered my mother's baffled eye roll as she picked up a trainer, ran her finger along the mouselike suede, then returned to whatever she was doing.

Somehow things had changed. These days I understood the joy of a new pair of running shoes and what they represented.

I started making up random queries so I could call my dad

for a pep talk from time to time. He was becoming more than a father and more than a friend; he was becoming a genuine inspiration.

As the training runs became longer, I started doing more of them near my parents' house in Wiltshire. Aside from the glorious views, there were the benefits of my dad's advice. We enjoyed marking out potential courses on his chaotically photocopied Ordnance Survey maps the night before, drawing the route with a highlighter and then wrapping the paper in a plastic folder that I could carry in my palm. I'd be approaching a hill that had appeared so inviting from the comfort of a gliding car's window but was in fact a relentless, demonic gradient on foot. Just when I was about to lose hope, he'd pull up alongside me with water and half a banana. "I figured you'd be about here!" he'd say as I tearfully asked to be driven home. "Not a chance," he'd say. "I saw the way you took that hill on, you've got at least three more miles in your legs. See you later for lunch!"

It was like talking to a hellish tower of confidence. There was no negotiating his faith in what I could achieve. At times infuriating, it was also powerful. It kept me going. It got me home in time for lunch.

I was also calling my brother more often, and for increasingly geeky conversations: maps, routes, training schedules, lined socks, and weird new food groups. We learned about an interval training method called the fartlek and giggled at the name.

By Christmas I was a proper runner. I received thermal running tights from my brother on Christmas Day and didn't break my marathon-training schedule. Running was changing everything.

It wasn't just my family who saw changes in me and my

attitude. After a lifetime of endlessly discussing feelings, having spats, and indulging in gossip with my mother, sister, and female friends, I recognized that I was developing confidence and a better understanding of how to communicate. Emotions didn't always need to be spelled out or talked to death. Sometimes time is how you spend your love. Without ever expressing our newfound closeness, I realized that as the time I spent with my father and brother had increased, so had my confidence when dealing with men in general.

After Christmas, marathon training continued, and I started garnering—maybe even commanding—more respect from those around me. I enjoyed having my body praised for what it could do rather than how it looked. For years I felt my male friends had seen me as a woman first and a friend second, and I had never troubled a boyfriend with my almost anti-competitive spirit. My newfound physical ease didn't merely translate to moving my arse closer to the holy grail of looking better in jeans but to making the world seem smaller, more accessible, on foot. It became—and remains—a delicious pleasure to stride up the escalator in a tube station, my breathing steady and the strength of my legs powering me.

It wasn't only moments of passing smugness that were my treats; it was being able to have more fun with more spontaneity. I will never forget the look on my toddler godson's face when I saw him for the first time in a few weeks and picked him up like a tiny rocket ship, blasting him into the air. After months of running up hills, my arms were stronger than I had realized, and my enthusiastic "Woooooosh!" was followed by my nearly shoving him through the kitchen ceiling. We laughed conspiratorially as we both realized that I'd surprised myself with my new strength.

Whenever anyone asked me how I'd done it, the answer was simple: I decided to be able to.

As my body changed and my sense of its capabilities started to shift, I developed a more masculine side to my personality and, dare I say it, a competitive streak. I was getting to know my way around London per mile rather than per tube stop. I was happy to engage in sporting chat in a way that I could have done only with a heavy sense of irony before. Just as I had relied on goofing around on the sports field to mask anxieties I'd felt about performing sport, I had become dependent on humor when discussing it as well. Before, wry comments about "men chasing a ball around a field" were as far as I could get where sports were concerned, and I was the first to leap in with "Yeah, I can do a marathon too. A *brunch* marathon" when the London Marathon was televised on a Sunday morning every April. Now I wanted to chat about it. And I was finding it easier to spot—and then ignore—others who were relying on the same humor mechanisms instead of engaging with the subject. In time, I found the confidence to breezily wander around shops filled with fitness gear.

My new knowledge and grit didn't lead to my becoming a social outcast; rather, people seemed more interested in me. While women were admiring of my tenacity with training and my ever leaner legs, men wanted to know more about me. I was garnering admiration, interest, and kudos not just from blokes I was dating but those I'd known for years. My male friends were viewing me with renewed respect: *She's actually going through with this,* I could see them thinking.

My confidence filtered into my relationships with female friends too. I sensed respect from them: I was sticking to my plan, I was going to get it done. In embracing my masculine side, I was becoming a better woman. I found it easier to admit that I had goals or dreams and that it took dedication to achieve them.

After a lifetime of accepting that my body was to be looked at rather than used, I was learning to appreciate what it could do. Food became a practicality, not merely an indulgence or a torment; I came to associate it with fuel. I never stopped enjoying it, but I enjoyed it differently—because it helped me, not because I had guiltily used it as a bribe to get me through bleak days or cold nights. I became proud of my strong thighs. I didn't care that I would never be as thin as some girls. I knew I would be stronger than many. While compliments are always lovely, I struggled to care when people remarked on how much weight I'd lost. "But have you seen what I can do now?" was all I ever wanted to reply.

My perspective on exercise shifted. It was no longer about getting fit or reaching aesthetic perfection. Now I was enjoying the thrill of setting goals and sticking to them, of developing the kind of mental discipline only sports could inspire. I saw that competitiveness and sweat needn't be unfeminine or aggressive qualities. They could be attractive.

My goals and challenges weren't all Pollyanna-ish either. I cherished the simple childlike glee of shoving on weird, bright stretchy clothes and going outside to leap around to loud music. I let my mind float off, pretending to be whichever rock star I was listening to, or imagining I was running from certain peril, or simply that I was winning a race I'd never entered. I chuckled inwardly as I wondered if passersby could see me nodding to a particularly juicy bass line. I felt my face soften as a song appeared on my playlist that had been sent to me as part of a flirtation. I grinned as a song that reminded me of a particularly high-octane party appeared out of nowhere. I was getting little extra bursts of living out there with my music, the intensity of each emotion heightened by the fast pumping of my blood.

My confidence, which in the past had been battered and bruised by romantic and career endeavors, felt as if it had been given emotional Botox. Boosted from within, it felt plumped up, more delicious than it had in years. Running around meant that I saw more people, my place in the world felt a little sturdier, everything felt a little less of a catastrophe and a bit more like the natural ebb and flow of life. It became harder to scuttle home from a bad meeting or an awkward date, head bowed over my phone or a magazine, then stay in and sulk for a weekend: There was a running plan to be dealt with. I couldn't stay in, or marathon day would catch me out. Once I was out of the house, I felt my gaze shift outward again. A granny struggling with some shopping that I could help with, my arms stronger now. A couple squabbling on a park bench, reminding me that being in a couple wasn't an automatic pass to happiness. And then the warmth of a bath and the sofa as a reward, rather than the fetidness of having been in one or the other for forty-eight hours.

Running ceased to be about what others might see when they looked at me. It became about what I saw when I ran. I started to find the change in the seasons more interesting than the changes in my body. This weight was the heaviest I could have shed. I was no longer running to prove that I could finish a marathon, or to impress my dad, or to sound good on dates. I was using these runs to give me clarity and focus, to remind myself of what I was capable of, and to spur me on in all areas of my life. I felt unstoppable.

Until one day I had to stop.

5

Injury

Everyone who has run knows that its most important value is in removing tension and allowing release from whatever other cares the day may bring.

—Jimmy Carter

I knew it would be a cold January run when I set out from home to Hampstead Heath. I had on my new thermal leggings and a pair of gloves. After half an hour, I was coping pretty well. The tip of my nose was as ruddy as ever, but my eyes were not watering too much, and my feet were surprisingly warm. For reasons I didn't fully understand, my hips were taking the full blast of the afternoon's icy winds. Each stride felt more like a stinging slap than the last. It had happened once or twice before, but the winter had been long and cold, and I assumed that this was just a weak spot of mine.

Stopping to cross the street, I tried lifting my heel up behind me and grabbing my foot to stretch out my hip flexors. I slapped the tops of my thighs on either side, trying to get the blood circulating, anything to warm up. It was no use; the pain was getting worse. Eventually, I decided that I wouldn't run as far as I had planned and headed home with only two thirds of the run completed. I had to almost drag my leg behind me, despondent at the parade of runners sailing by.

An hour later, once I'd had a hot bath and changed, the pain across the top of my right leg was still excruciating. It felt as if someone had tightened the ligaments and tendons holding me together. I wanted to stretch and stretch, though it never made anything feel any better.

I headed out to the tube, on my way to meet a friend at the cinema. I barely made it to the station, almost unable to lift my leg. By the time I reached the South Bank, tears of pain were stinging my eyes. What had happened? I hadn't fallen or knocked myself. I hadn't knowingly sprained anything. I had no idea what could be causing such piercing agony, and I spent the length of the film shifting in my seat, longing to know if a decent rest would ease it. As the credits rolled, I dreaded standing.

Within forty-eight hours, I was sitting in a physical therapist's consulting room. I was lucky to have been recommended a decent sports therapist. Josie—a dark-haired woman as tiny as she was commanding—was sympathetic and genuinely interested in what was causing my pain. In minutes she had got me down to my underpants and bra and had stuck tiny dots—the sort that usually indicate that a painting has been sold—on my shoulders, hips, elbows, and the backs of my knees. Then she put me on a running machine and told me to jog, which she filmed for a few minutes. The hip pain had eased considerably by then, but I was still wincing.

Once I was dressed, Josie rewound the footage and looked at it. Then we watched it together, her gaze hard with concentration, mine glazed with the sort of hopeful ignorance I used to reserve for trying to spot the baby in a friend's ultrasound snapshot. Moments later, Josie looked at me and asked, "Have you had an accident recently that had a large impact on the left-hand side of your body?"

I had not.

"And possibly a secondary impact on the right?"

Nothing rang any bells. I had been fine for months, perhaps a year. Sure, I often had pain in my pelvis after sitting down for long journeys, and had done since long before I started running, but it seemed like a fair trade-off for a job that saw me mostly sitting at a laptop or curled in bizarre positions reading.

I gave her a blank look. "No, nothing."

"Are you sure? You seem to have sustained a pretty big blow," Josie repeated.

I racked my brain. Surely I would remember a massive blow to the left-hand side of my body. "No, really, I'm fine."

"Okay, have you ever been in a traffic accident?" she persisted.

"Really, no, I have never been in a car crash," I replied, as frustration at her surety bubbled up in me.

As my mouth formed that final "sh," the realization hit me with a crash of its own: Four years previously, I had been knocked off my Vespa on Kilburn High Road by an SUV when it turned right without looking and drove straight into me. Sure, I had never been in a car crash. That was because I had been on a scooter. And then in the air.

As I watched the tape replay again and again, every bit of pain I had felt for the last four years made sense. Josie slowed down the footage and showed me my running gait in motion, complete with all of its attendant weaknesses. At the time of the accident, I had been checked over and told that, aside from a few ripped muscles, I had sustained no serious injuries. Back then I wasn't a runner. What was more than evident as I watched myself run on the treadmill, the little dots rising and falling in irregular patterns, was that I had been injured after all. My pelvis was not in the correct place; it had been knocked around by the impact of that huge vehicle. Consequently, my body had adapted around the injury, growing weaker and stronger in equal measure.

My running training had made me stronger, but not symmetrically so. I had started to develop something of an imbalanced Frankenstein's monster of a body. The front of one thigh was strong with a weak hamstring behind it. The reverse was true of the other leg, which was slightly farther forward than its partner on account of my misaligned pelvis. The pattern was repeating itself across my entire body, until my front hip flexor was no longer able to pull my leg forward without excruciating pain. All because one woman in a Chelsea Tractor could not be bothered to check her side mirrors four years ago.

I sat on the edge of Josie's consulting couch, watching my marathon dream fade to tatters. I swallowed time and again, desperate not to cry in front of someone I had just met. What was to be done? Could I run again? Or were all of those people who had claimed that running would "destroy your legs" correct after all?

Josie calmly talked me through what I had to do and how we were going to get it sorted. Part of me had been hoping for something high-tech, a properly medical problem that could be remedied with a prescription. The reality was much the same as most of my running journey: Hard work was required. She told me immediately that I could not run for at least a month, until I had done exercises every day to strengthen and rebalance the muscle groups working so hard against each other. I began a daily regimen of painstaking Pilates-like movements—often while tied to a door handle or the back of a chair with stretchy physio banding to get the necessary resistance. Slowly, over the next few weeks, I managed to right myself. Though it was too late for me to be perfect in time for the marathon, the dream was not over. I submitted to whatever Josie instructed me, secretly impressed that I had endured the pain as long as I had.

It wasn't the pain or the tedium of the exercises that proved to be the worst part of the experience. It was not being able to run. Under Josie's instruction, I joined my local gym for a month so that I could keep my fitness up on other machines. Anything but running. What so recently had been an activity that filled me with sheer dread was now what I longed to do more than anything else. I felt caged in the gym.

I would wake having dreamed of running, and in my waking hours, I fretted endlessly about what would happen the next time I attempted a run. The idea that I once was anxious about buying a pair of socks seemed ludicrous compared to my fears about giving up running for good. Having gone from viewing my body as a tedious accessory to something genuinely useful, I now saw it as a great treasure. For six weeks I followed Josie's orders; I shunned high heels; I prayed for the best.

With running injuries, it is often the case that you don't know how recovered you are until you undertake a long run. Though you have to be prepared to fail, you can't let yourself consider that tiny window of possibility. As in a grim game of chicken, I vacillated between wanting as many people as possible to know about the injury and keeping it a secret so it couldn't take hold and gain power over me.

As marathon day grew closer, I began some tentative recovery runs. Amazingly, the pain had gone. It looked as if I would be on the starting blocks after all. I never managed to catch up with my original training plan, but I did what I could within the limited time frame. I got through March, thanks to Josie, late nights spent chatting on the London Marathon website, and a steady stream of texts, e-mails, and chats with my dad. I stretched, I fretted, I did my strengthening exercises. I watched the entire first season of *The Wire* standing with one foot tied to the bottom of a table leg. I did everything I could think of to get through, up to and including pestering everyone I knew for sponsorship, in order to drive home how much I needed to get round that course. One fact remained: The only way to find out if I was physically—or mentally—capable of finishing a marathon was to try and run a marathon.

6

The London Marathon

*If you are losing faith in human nature, go out
and watch a marathon.*

–Kathrine Switzer

I could not have done more to prepare for my first London
Marathon, yet I have never been less prepared for anything
in my life. My mental image of the starting blocks was not dis
similar to that of an egg-and spoon race at a school sports day:
a handful of eager enthusiasts willing to give it their very best.
The reality felt more like the chaos of a music festival. I was
exhausted before I reached the starting line.

The day before, my parents and sister came up to London to
cheer me and my brother along. We all went to the local pub for
a high-carb lunch. I walked delicately, worried that the slightest knock could damage my chances of reaching the finish line
with a misplaced bruise or sprain. I did not eat delicately; I pol-
ished off a bowl of seafood pasta as if it were my death-row
meal. Then my sister ordered us shots of sambuca, convincing
us that it would wear off long before bedtime.

Before I went to bed, I checked my sports bag, all packed for the next morning, and laid out my running gear next to it. When bedtime arrived, I found myself wishing for more sambuca. I had never been more awake. Perhaps it was nerves, perhaps it was my body swimming in carbohydrates. Either way, I slept lightly, lying awkwardly in a variety of positions that I thought would rest my muscles as much as possible, while a million worst-case scenarios painted my mind in Technicolor.

Within seconds of my alarm sounding, I was whipping up scrambled eggs with a speed and focus that would have made my military father proud. I swallowed them grimly, still full from the day before. Their relentless rubberiness reminded me of school food: necessary nutrition and nothing more. I dressed, checked my bag another six or seven times, and sat on the very edge of the sofa, waiting for the taxi. Twenty minutes later, I was approaching Charing Cross station to meet my brother. His training had gone more smoothly, but he was just as nervous as I was. We had shared late-night anxieties, bizarre and hitherto unfamiliar food cravings, and endless tips, and he had provided a steadfast level of support since day one. I could barely wait to see him.

I had imagined he'd be easy to spot, a lone nerdy runner in a swarm of London day-trippers and homeward-bound nightclubbers. The reality made me draw breath. The *only* passengers at Charing Cross were runners, a sea of tense, solitary figures in wicking fabric. Eventually his face appeared in the swarm. There was barely space for us all on the trains heading toward Greenwich, and we shuffled onto the carriages in eerie silence. I assumed everyone else was an old-timer, destined for an impressive three-hour finish time and a quick fry-up before heading home. I know better now: That silence was a result of us all thinking the same thing. Everyone was nervous, whatever their fitness or experience.

We poured out of the station at Blackheath and began the fifteen-minute walk across the grass. The weather reports had been mixed all week, predicting everything from rain and wind to sun and unicorns. As we headed through southeast London, the air was crisp and clear. I imagined I had joined a cult that met in a secret London. We were marching to some sort of promised land, searching for answers from a leader we had yet to meet. It was an hour before the official start time; what would we do until then? What else did this strange pilgrimage hold for us? The answer, it turned out, was Porta-Potties.

My brother and I made two stops, thoughts of roadside peeing looming larger in our terrified minds. On entering and exiting, we avoided eye contact with the other runners, kindred pilgrims complicit in the same fleeting madness.

When we reached the starting-line area, the atmosphere became more like that of a carnival or feast day than the earlier reverence. Thick black speakers belted out relentless motivational music. A cheesy DJ read dedications and good-luck messages. A gospel choir would not have surprised me. Half an hour later, I spotted one.

It was an enormous spectacle, and we were irredeemably a part of it. Numbed by the volume of activity around me, I handed over my bag with barely a second thought.

Relieved not to have missed any trains or broken any legs en route, my brother and I became almost hysterical, the mood of the crowd sweeping us up in nervous anticipation. Nibbling on crackers and bananas, we joined the hordes of runners leaning against trees doing last-minute stretches, and took silly photos of each other in our running vests. Maybe it would be fun after all, we started to tell each other, glancing around. Everyone seemed to be okay. I relaxed into the idea of spending the day in Greenwich Park, getting to know my new friends, my fellow pilgrims. Then, suddenly, we were called to the starting enclosures. Just as suddenly, I desperately wanted to go home.

Runners at the London Marathon line up by expected finish times. The fastest runners leave first so they don't get trapped behind the rest of us—the nervous, the slow, and the becostumed. I was divided into a pen based on my anticipated time, as predicted six months earlier on the application. The me who had filled in that form now seemed as foreign as the professional athletes warming up for the BBC cameras. I'd had no idea what I might be capable of; the prospect of finishing had filled me with wide-eyed wonder. Consequently, I had no recollection of what I had stated as my predicted time back in October, and it was only when we collected our race numbers that I discovered I'd gone for the slowest time possible. My brother, who had done some basic research, had not. He was due in a pen two hundred meters away. He turned and grinned at me. "Good luck!" he said, stretching his arms out for a hug and doing his best to mask his own nerves. "You'll probably win!"

My baby brother, heading off without me. My bottom lip wobbled. "Have an amazing time," I replied, trying not to look flustered by the huge number of runners flocking toward the starting enclosures. "See you at the end—and text me when you've finished!"

I walked toward my pen, which seemed to be populated by the elderly and people dressed as cartoon characters. My cheeks burned with shame as I realized that my low expectations for myself had labeled me as one of this lot. I looked around and smiled, hoping for a similarly aged face that might take pity

on me and smile back. Everyone else seemed to be with someone, bonding over something. The crowd packed in around
me, emphasizing the aching loneliness that washed over me. I
felt something like the homesickness that I had felt as an eight-
year-old at boarding school for the first time. The thought of the
run no longer bothered me. But the thought of doing it alone,
with nothing but my thoughts for the next few hours, flooded
me with anxiety.

Another problem I had never even considered was creeping up on me—my fear of crowds. I have never been to a music
festival; I avoid big sales at the mall; and I skulk around at the
beginnings and ends of big sporting events until almost everyone has left. I have jumped fences in Hyde Park and run through
the trees in the dark to avoid the drunken crowds coming out
of concerts. I always, always seek to avoid my worst nightmare:
being caught up in an unpredictable tsunami of humans. If possible, I will walk rather than take a packed train, or I'll wait until
a crowd has passed, so horrified am I of being moved by a mass
of bodies in a direction I can't control.

I looked around the pens, occasionally bouncing on tip-
toes to check on the river of people ahead, and saw that this
was exactly where I was. Six months of training, most of them
entirely alone, for this: the biggest crowd I had ever been part
of. As I had pounded my local pavements alone, run across ox
droves and through grassy valleys circling my parents' home,
and around the lanes of Tobago on holiday, I had never considered the glaringly obvious fact that on the day there would
be other runners alongside me. How had I not thought of that?
How would I find my place among the bodies? How would I
deal with the relentless lava flow of runners?

My heart hammered in my chest, and I stared down at my

shoes, hoping to contain the rising panic. The feet around me began their slow shuffle toward the start line. I looked up; the red start banner was so far away that we could barely see it. We moved forward, the chatter rising and falling, people wishing one another good luck. The pace quickened as we turned the corner and suddenly saw the arch, with its familiar clock sitting above it. The crowd began to jog, slowly, apprehensively, at first. And then a real run as we crossed the mats that triggered the timer chips tied to our shoes. People around me cheered and whooped as they set off. I let out a nervous, fluttering laugh. I was running a marathon.

Five minutes into the first mile, the crowd had eased into a steady pace. I was able to overtake a few slow joggers. We were heading through Greenwich, streets of smart residential houses with families outside—many still in pajamas—wishing the runners well and cheering them along as they hugged morning cups of tea. Their smiles lifted me as my heart rate leveled out and my feet found a regular rhythm.

Half an hour later, my attitude to the crowd had shifted. I felt dependent on the steady thud of others' feet as we curled gently round corners as one, our pulses quickening in unison as we headed up the occasional inclines. I looked around and started to recognize faces, numbers, and names from earlier in the day. We were like a family now. I would not complete this alone after all. A surge of confidence bubbled up in me, and I began grinning and waving at the spectators. I felt like a rock star, as though an occasional glance from me could inspire a watching child to a lifetime of athletic prowess. *Yes! You can be whomever you want to be!* I felt like shrieking it to each and every one of them as I sailed past, legs strong and heart pumping.

We turned another corner, and I spotted a line of children

with their hands outstretched, hoping to catch high fives from the passing competitors. They went largely ignored, as the crowd was shuffling for positions, teddy bears jostling among Smurfs for superiority on the road. Occasionally, someone would run by and slap the children's hands, leaving a little ripple of grins behind them. I decided I wanted to do that. I spotted a gap in the sea of people and took a couple of steps toward the edge of the road, stretching out my arm. I was yearning for a bit of human contact, and these small hands seemed like the perfect comfort and acknowledgment.

I leaned forward, reaching out for one of the hands and continuing to run as I grinned down at the child. I felt the ground rushing up toward me. Before I could work out what was happening, my left hip struck the pavement, and a rush of heat seared across my thigh as I skidded along the road. I had not spotted the curb; in reaching for those hands, I had lost my footing and fallen, my legs a rag-doll jumble. I stared at the tarmac, sweating under the disappointed gaze of the children, painfully aware of the inconvenience I was causing other runners, as they had to step around me. Gasping, I sprang up, pushed my hair off my face, and carried on running.

I longed for the debilitating shame of tripping and falling alone, when all that is left for you to do is glare at the guilty pavement. I had done that many times and almost developed a technique for coping with it. This shame was a hundred times worse, surrounded as I was by an audience. Their pitying gasps, their shaking heads, their angry shuffles past.

The price of vanity, I could feel them thinking. *Only a first-timer would do that.*

Soon the pain of embarrassment was replaced by a rush of physical pain. Each time my right thigh rose toward me, I saw my shredded running tights. I was grazed and bruised from shoulder to elbow to knuckles, as well as the length of my thigh, where flecks of lacerated Lycra were embedded. The blood from my leg was starting to drip down, and my pelvis was giving off its familiar dull ache.

Sweat met blood met fabric in dappled crops of stinging. Each step caused the fissures on my thigh to crackle and split, and a fresh smattering of pain worked its way across me. I knew I had to get some antiseptic on the grazes. A mile later, I spotted an ambulance tent. I ran off the main road and into the tent. I arrived, panting, unused to a world where I stood still and others moved. A reassuring-looking elderly lady with a whipped-cream topping of a hairdo looked up and smiled at me. "Hello, dear. Our first customer of the day! What seems to be the problem?" she asked with all the urgency of a woman judging a sponge cake at a town fair. The feet passing outside the tent made a constant rumble as all the runners I had overtaken in the last hour steadily passed me. "Oh dear, that's a nasty graze, isn't it?" Her tone was one of a kindly grandmother.

I'm running a race! I wanted to shout. *Help me, I need to get back there.* One of the Smurfs passed the tent's entrance as it flapped open in the breeze.

"Pam, do we have any antiseptic wipes?"

My heart was struggling to know what to do: beat slower because I was standing still or beat faster in panic at my new friend's apparent lack of urgency.

"Oooh, I think they're in the hold-all that June brought in," came the reply.

"Now, dear, can you just fill in this form so they know what we've done with you?"

"I wanted you to check there was no grit in my grazes, really."

"I understand, dear. Now, what's your date of birth?"

"The fourteenth of—"

"Oh, now isn't that lovely eye makeup, June? So nice that the young lady's made an effort for the big day . . ."

I wanted to be angry, but I was so relieved that someone was taking care of me. I wanted to be running, but there was no chance of that for another few minutes, at least.

"Apparently, the weather's going to turn in a bit, but you wouldn't believe it, looking at the sky, would you?"

I winced: I'll never know if it was the pain of her dabbing at the grazes or the sight of two men dressed as rhinoceros stomp past the tent. It had taken me three minutes to get past them half an hour ago.

Eventually, June's friend deemed me fit to run. I begged for some anti-inflammatory pills for the bruising, but they were firm—they were not allowed to give me any. I left the tent and my twelve minutes of unscheduled static contemplation behind me. Rejoining the throng was harder than starting at the beginning of the race. I had been wrenched in the wrong direction; all my confidence had evaporated, and I was surrounded by a gaggle of fancy-dress runners, valiant old folk, and others barely doing more than a walk. I loved these guys; I knew I could happily spend the next five hours with them and trundle to the finish, declaring myself injured. I also knew how hard I had trained. And I knew my injuries were probably superficial. I had to make a decision: run around them in order to regain a steady pace, getting a few miles under my belt, or run treacle-slow, expending no energy on dodging rhinos but letting the marathon continue almost infinitely. To make matters worse, the thud of pain was reappearing, and it was only going to get worse.

I chose the former, and I didn't enjoy a second of it. Instead of running in a straight line, I was effectively running twice as fast and far as everyone around me. I wove across the road, shimmying between women chatting about their grandchildren, ducking beneath wacky headgear, and dodging around Mr. Men. Every twist and shimmy created blooms of pain in my joints while I seemed to go nowhere. The heavens finally opened, just as the reports had been promising. I was glad for the rain, as it hid the tears I shed for three miles. As I plodded through the rain, my shoes swelled, and my heart felt as heavy as my sodden ponytail. I was playing out different excuses in my mind, performing imaginary role-plays of how I'd explain to friends and family that I'd given up on the marathon halfway because of some grazes and sprains.

This reverie had become almost enjoyable, the masochism of my new determination to fail consuming me, when my phone buzzed with a text from my father. They were nearby, under a mile away, waiting to cheer me on up Jamaica Road, around mile eleven. My father, my mother, and my sister. I refreshed my master plan. I would keep going at least until I had seen them; it would be rude to deprive them of the chance to see me running after waiting all that time. Then I would decide whether to abandon the mission. As I approached, I started to crane my neck, hoping to spot one of them in the thick ropes of the crowd, maybe catch a smile. No need. I heard my mother's voice rise like a lark above the rest of the uniform cheering: "COME ON, MY DARLING GIRL, YOU ARE DOING SO WELL, NOT TOO FAR BEHIND YOUR BROTHER! KEEP GOING, YOU STRONG, STRONG THING, AND MAYBE YOU'LL CATCH HIM AND SHOW THOSE BOYS WHAT WE'RE MADE OF!"

"I've fallen!" I replied, pointing to my shredded leggings.

"KEEP GOING, YOU LAUGH IN THE FACE OF PAIN!"

was the reply I received, amid further whooping from the three of them.

A concerned woman on the sidelines edged her stroller away from my raucous family. I shrieked, as did my sister when she saw me, and they all burst into cheering, waving, and clapping. Their fellow onlookers understood that a loved one had been spotted and joined in with the yelling. A ripple of goodwill passed through them and made its way toward me and my neighboring runners. Someone nearby slapped me on the back as I passed.

Whether you know them or not, supporters make an incalculable difference when you are running a race. Cheers are never, ever unwelcome. (Unless, perhaps, the cheerers are enjoying a cigarette with their roadside pint and blowing the smoke into the runners' faces.) Those few seconds of hearing people shout your name can keep a lonely runner going for miles.

As we turned along the river and approached Tower Bridge and the thirteen-mile mark, I felt part of a communal effort once again. The mass of runners hugged against me as the road narrowed and the towers loomed into sight. The bands and cheering grew louder. A communal energy spurred us on and we were all grinning. We felt like superheroes as we crossed the river. The sun broke through the clouds and dried us out, making us giddy with glee. I grinned at a Captain Caveman roaring and waving his plastic club at the spectators. He caught my eye and grinned back. My earlier resentment of the slower runners had dissipated. I felt that we were in it together. We were doing it for each other. And we were halfway! Maybe I could do it after all, and maybe, *maybe,* it was worth it.

After Tower Bridge, the marathon route heads toward the city, and for about a mile the road is divided in two with runners going in both directions. Those at thirteen miles are heading east, and adjacent to them are the runners already at twenty-two miles, heading for the final stretch. It serves as an almost immediate reality check after the rock-star high of crossing the river. Where minutes ago you felt like an iconic athlete, capable of anything, here you are confronted with a stampede of runners nine miles ahead of you. It was exactly as I hit this point that "halfway" ceased to sound like an achievement and became more of a punishment. I had to do this all over again? I had already been drenched, tearful, injured, ecstatic, and hysterical. Doing it a second time was absurd, out of the question, nonsense. Yet there seemed no alternative but to keep plodding on.

The crowd started to thin out as some runners slowed to a walk, others stopped to chat with loved ones or queue for a roadside toilet, and some dropped out altogether. The thundering mass that had crossed the bridge where the route was at its narrowest now spread across the wide avenues of the City of London. I could still see runners around me, but they were becoming fewer and fewer. There was no one close enough to talk to, no feet to stare at. There were barely any spectators. The space I had craved a couple of hours earlier now felt like a cruel echo chamber. I tried to convince myself that the end would appear soon.

Bereft of the iconic sights that we had passed earlier, feeling increasingly isolated and overtaken by tiredness, my mind began to play tricks on me. While my legs seemed able to keep going, my mental strength was collapsing. I began not just to doubt myself but to berate myself. *You're running around the City in a pair of ripped trousers to try and prove a point. You wouldn't be feeling like this if you had trained properly. All those runs where you didn't try your hardest because you were a bit tired, well, this is tiredness. You're weak because you're tired, you probably won't make it. You're weak even to be considering the fact that you won't make it. You're selfish, making your friends and family come and cheer for you when you're not that good. You're not tired, you're just lazy.*

The torrent of self-doubt continued for mile upon mile. The pain in my pelvis grew more acute. Soulless concrete and glass buildings dominated the landscape, growing taller as the route became more intricate between miles fifteen and twenty. The mile markers were out of sight and we were running in loops, weaving between huge office blocks that hid from view the next water station or cheering point. Just as I needed it most, my faith utterly vanished like a piece of tissue paper in flames.

Though I had devoted so much attention and preparation to avoiding hitting the physical Wall, I had devoted nothing to avoiding this emotional wall. No one had warned me about it, no one had told me how to prevent it, no one had prepared me for how to deal with it. Was I the only one feeling these things? Of course I assumed that I was, and I felt like the most pathetic runner of the pack. I would have been prepared to argue until sundown with anyone who had told me that I could do it. Even the most well-meaning roadside cheers were reaching my ears as jeers. I wanted to hide from them all, to conceal this certain humiliation. I was sure to the point of rage that this race was never going to end. For the first time all day, there was no doubt in my mind. It had nothing to do with nutrition, or tiredness, or hormones. Those were ludicrous suggestions. Mental doors suggesting any other possibility slammed shut the second I approached them. It was simple, I would be running forever.

I drew one final shred of inspiration from the sponsorship

money I had raised. As much as the training had been an epic journey, so had the fund-raising. My brother and I had contacted everyone we could think of, and set up a Facebook group tracking our progress in order to get as many people as possible following our mission and supporting it with donations.

I tried to replace the image I had of me weeping by the side of the road with the far more powerful images of the children I knew my friend Vanessa had worked with. I repeated to myself how much of a difference my contribution would make to them and their parents. I tried to remind myself—out loud at times— that my pain was temporary, whereas their hardships were permanent. When that didn't work, I tried to remember the good training days I'd had, to feel strong for the people I was running for, to achieve what they might never be able to. Then I texted my dad.

"Looks like I won't make it. Very weak now."

"Don't be ridiculous. Just tiredness. We are close."

"WHERE probably going to stop soon can't go on."

"BENEATH ONE CANADA SQUARE."

"What? We don't even go there."

"You do can see other runners now."

"Won't see you. Must have passed."

"What mile are you on? You will see us. The crowd is ready for you."

"Won't. Will probably just stop."

"KEEP GOING WE ARE NEAR."

That was it. I had missed them. They had traveled miles across central London to try and get to a second cheering, and it had been for nothing. My father probably had been staring at an unnecessary map as I passed, while my mother and sister gossiped. I bet they all saw my brother, who didn't need any support. Tears streamed down my face, and my pelvis creaked with pain. I resigned myself once again to the hopelessness of my cause as I rounded yet another corner to yet another tedious urban vista. Stupid bloody London.

I stared at my feet, grimly plodding forward. *Keep going, keep going,* I muttered to myself. I began to feel as if everyone around me was doing the same. I looked up. Everyone around me *was* doing the same. And there was my family, surrounded by a huge group of forty or fifty total strangers they seemed to have rallied to cheer when I appeared. "Keep going," they were yelling. "Keep going!"

Then I saw her, my mother, her hair balanced like a bird's nest, the result of too much excitement and too much weather. She seemed to have acclimated to the raucous crowds. My sister spotted me first, and the tears and giggles came together. My father was grinning widely. "I told you," he mouthed. I ran to the side of the road and flung myself at him for a hug. I felt my sister gingerly stroking my hair. Everyone around them carried on cheering, telling me I could make it, explaining how long they'd been waiting to see me and how much they had heard about my fall. My father placed his hand beneath my chin and lifted it to meet his gaze. "You will finish this. You have done the hardest part. You are strong."

I bleated about my pelvis, my tiredness, my despair. He wouldn't have it. He would not countenance the idea that I might not finish. There was no arguing with his calm granite faith. I hugged him again and rejoined the route. My legs remained exhausted, but my heart felt lighter. There was hope. I passed Captain Caveman's club, which had been discarded on the roadside among empty water bottles, and hoped he was feeling okay too. We began to weave away from the heart of the City, and the crowd seemed to get thicker again as the roads narrowed. I remembered one of the nuggets of advice my father had given my brother and me at lunch the previous day: Talk to someone if you get lonely. You don't have to run alone.

I felt a tap on my shoulder and turned round. A young man smiled at me and asked me to move aside. I did, confused by what seemed a very formal way to approach the simple step of overtaking someone. I saw two men behind him, bound to each other with the kind of wrist strap that I had only ever seen on toddlers in supermarkets. The older of the two men was blind, and the younger was leading him. The third man, who had tapped my shoulder, was clearing a path for them.

For a few hundred meters, I watched the team, marveling at how fit the third man must be to circle his team like that. I truly understood what running rings around someone meant as he raced about, covering twice their distance, alerting other runners to their approach with an effortless charm. It seemed easy to slot in behind them, watching the blind man's feet and using them as a pace guide while taking advantage of the small oasis of calm behind them. After half a mile, one of them offered me some of the sweets that they were eating. I took a cola bottle and thanked him profusely. The third man smiled and asked how I was getting on. I explained that my mood was clearing, but it had been dark for a while.

"It's a big deal, running a marathon," he reassured me, despite barely having broken a sweat and continuing to run rings around us.

"Is it your first time?" I asked timidly.

"No, this is our seventh."

"Wow, you've run seven marathons! All together?"

"Yes, we've done them in the last seven days."

"You've run . . . seven marathons in . . . seven days?"

"Yes, this is Blind Dave. He's doing it for charity."

My head was spinning. They had been doing this every day for a week. Yet they seemed like the sunniest people I'd encountered all day. I wanted to hug them but was reluctant to break their stride. So I ran alongside them for four or five miles, sharing food, water, and anecdotes. My father had been right. Just chatting distracted me from the excruciating pain in my hips and knees. Talking to them kept my mind busy, away from self-destructive and despairing monologues. And they reminded me how fleeting my own pain was. God knew how their hips and knees felt after seven marathons.

We headed away from the City and along the embankment to the final stretch. The crowds of spectators increased, and the cheering became frenzied. My grin was back. I was going to make it after all. I was looking around as the sites loomed into view. The river, the London Eye, the parks. I didn't care how my feet felt anymore. I knew I was going to make it.

"You look like you're perking up," said my new running pal. "You should speed up for the last mile, do it in style. But make sure you enjoy it."

So I did.

A final desperate surge of energy bubbled up and propelled me faster, away from Blind Dave and his helpers. Everything I had felt at the eighteen-mile point flipped into reverse. Every single training run made sense as my legs found the power to overtake handfuls of other runners while I grinned and waved at the onlookers. I wasn't a failure, I wasn't pathetic, I wasn't weak. I had proved that I could set a goal and meet it. I had shown that I could redefine who I was and who I could be.

I had discovered that tenacity in myself along with a huge well of goodwill in my friends and loved ones.

I was literally following in my father's footsteps. I was driven by his faith in me, in the texts I'd received all day from him and others. I was riding a tide of adrenaline, doing it for all of them. I saw children catching sight of their loved ones and felt proud of everyone around me. My legs were getting stronger as we approached Big Ben and then curved toward the Mall. I was a tourist attraction, a superhero, a medal winner.

The finish line seemed to be coming toward me as every part of my body heaved with the final effort and an all-consuming relief that I was about to cross the line. As I approached it, there was only one thought in my mind: *I am never, ever doing this again.* My feet carried me over the line, and I threw my hands above my head to look up at the red banner. That thought was immediately replaced by another: *Next time I could do it faster.*

7

The London Marathon.
Again

In running it doesn't matter if you come in first,
in the middle of the pack, or last. You can say
"I have finished." There is a lot of satisfaction in that.

—Fred Lebow, New York City marathon cofounder

I glided through the summer after my first marathon basking in the shimmery golden rays of my victory. At business
meetings, at weddings, at Sunday lunches, people who hadn't
seen me in a while wanted to catch up on every detail of my
impossible feat. How on earth had I managed it? How had I
trained? How had I discovered I could do such a thing? I was
the Girl Who Did, an inspiration to all!

I was convinced I'd be a runner for life. I was high on my
achievement and thrilled by others' fascination. I glowed when
my friends sought my running advice; I gave it freely. People
nodded thoughtfully as I blessed them with my knowledge,
while I was intrigued by how obvious it usually was. The only

answer I had for those who said they would never be able to make it farther than 5K was: "You have to decide to. You just have to want to." That was all I had done. I had wanted to.

Somewhere in my subconscious, something was shifting. A tide was receding. An opaqueness was settling over my marathon glow. I started to refer to my running self as another self, a temporary self, a self who had been built to make an impact, not to withstand one. I heard myself referring to what I had done rather than what I did. A subtle resignation to that experience being an exceptional time in my life seemed to settle in. I was not a runner—I had run.

The act of running returned to being something hypothetical: something that celebrities did to sell DVDs, something that shallow people tormented themselves with in order to stay slim, something that others did with élan while I pottered along with my handbag and a Twix bar. As for the psychological side, it must have been something I'd made up. It felt like a fad, like the time that I decided to study homeopathy, or the year I spent convinced that Simon Cowell was sexy.

I had never imagined that it would all go away as fast as I had created it, if not faster. I was exhausted, and the thought of running was repulsive to me. The sports gear I had chosen so carefully seemed as alien as a school uniform. Once so familiar it was now merely representative of a bygone stage in my life. I thought I had become a runner. I had just become someone who could run a marathon. I didn't know how different the two were back then.

Within a year of finishing that first London Marathon, I was no longer running. Perhaps I was making it round the park once a month, but I was getting progressively less fit, less healthy, and less happy. I had done a marathon; why did I need to run anymore? The motivation had deserted me. My toenails grew back, and with them a layer of extra me. My muscles softened, my heart slowed, and my skin grew dull again. I focused on other things—I changed my work situation; I moved from London to Brighton, a seafront city on the south coast about forty-five minutes on the train from London; and I made new friends.

That first summer living in Brighton I was exhausted, unhealthy, and heartbroken. I had started smoking again and felt ashamed when I saw London friends who associated me with a swooshing ponytail and a pair of running shoes. There was one remaining thread of healthiness that kept me going: the seafront. As I had done three years previously, I walked myself happy. I left my flat, still mesmerized by the fact that I lived with the sea on my doorstep, and headed either east or west along the coast. I walked everywhere, down the hill to the seafront, along the beach to wherever I needed to be, and then back up. The rest of my new home went largely unexplored.

Then, with a lightning bolt, everything changed. A friend needed me. My pal Julia, who had been so utterly steadfast in her support over my horrible summer, asked me to run the London Marathon with her. One of her dearest friends had died suddenly from a particularly aggressive form of cancer, weeks after his diagnosis, and left Julia and their social circle crippled with shock and grief. Julia, who had a toddler at home and was utterly devastated, was overwhelmed by the need to do something with her pain. She had to pay tribute, create some good from the suffering, do something that would make her friend proud.

Julia is not a woman who makes false promises or asks idle favors. One of my most inspiring can-do friends, she had long been the one I turned to for undiluted real talk when things were hard. She was always the first to tell me when a boyfriend was "good for nothing beyond giving you wet shoulders," her expression for men who ended up weeping on me. She never hesitated to encourage me to take career risks. She was strong. So to see her weakened was not just upsetting but profoundly unusual. It convinced me that anything really is possible. For her to pull through something that could make her seem so frail, she would need every scrap of help I could give her.

I had become completely accustomed to saying I would never run the London Marathon again: I would never earn a bib, I would never find the time to train, and I would never be that young again. These weren't excuses; I genuinely believed them. If there was no need, why should I do it? Now there was need.

"It doesn't matter if we walk it," Julia said. "I just need someone to be there with me, someone who knows what it's all like."

When someone you love has experienced a tragedy, you cannot say no to anything that might ease her grief. Committing to help Julia run in memory of her dear friend Jerome was a decision I didn't hesitate over. Seeing her visible pain created a rush of "What's the worst that could happen? My toes might hurt, but that's it." It hadn't been that bad, had it?

Before I knew it, I was going to run my second marathon, and on top of that, I was helping another person through it. Now I had to convince someone else that she could run, that she would finish, that it would be worth it. We committed to raising a large amount of money for the Institute of Cancer Research, and then we started training—Julia in London, me in Brighton. Our online communication was constant, with me explaining everything from basic training plans to what highs and lows Julia could expect to feel after runs. In return, she was always there when I texted her "Help it's raining here give me a funny reason to leave the sofa." A reply never failed to follow moments later.

A huge fear that once dogged me had lifted for one simple reason: I knew what to expect. I knew what the emotional dips were and where they were likely to come. I knew what it felt like to need the loo on a long run and to overcome it (or not). And I knew with absolute certainty that I could finish a marathon.

I also remembered that I had grown up in an environment where my parents engaged in feats of endurance without fanfare. My father's marathon prowess gave him the authority to tell me with zero hesitation that I could run that first marathon. My mother's family is from Trinidad—veterans of carnival. And what is carnival if not a marathon: two days spent on your feet wearing bright skimpy clothes, sweating profusely as you tread and retread the streets of the capital while people hand you sugary drinks. What was more, I'd had one of the greatest tools that a first-time marathoner can get her hands on: a support system, people around me who had absolute faith that I would finish, even if I did not believe it myself. I was determined to give the same kind of support to Julia, who was bigger than I was and even less sporty. She was going to need it.

The training started well. My confidence-building campaign was working, and Julia made incredible (if not literal) leaps. In a matter of weeks, she transformed from a woman who thought that the idea of her getting round the park was hilarious, to one who could confidently complete five kilometers half walking, half running, then one who could run the whole way. Best of all, she seemed to be enjoying it. Having spent the last year or so at home looking after her little boy, she relished the little pockets of space in her day that running created. She could clear her head and lose herself in the post-run endorphins. She realized that running with a hangover was not the worst thing on earth, and it often got rid of a hangover altogether. Her confidence, so shaken by grief, started to return. Her cheeks began to glow. Julia was back.

Meanwhile, in Brighton I was reacquainting myself with the idea of running, not to mention running itself. I had agreed to take part in this epic mission without hesitation and with little or no consideration of what it would mean for me. My only reservation was not that I might not finish it but that the relentlessness of training would bore me on the second go. Compared to London's parks, hills, and back streets, my beloved Brighton seafront seemed rather limiting. One of the greatest joys of my previous marathon training had been the huge variety of landscape I'd encountered: cemeteries, narrow seventeenth-century streets, wide sloping Regency terraces, the wilds of Hampstead Heath. Now my runs would have the same two views for the next six months: You go one way and you see the Palace Pier or the marina. You go the other and you see the West Pier and Shoreham power station.

Except that wasn't what happened at all. The view was never the same, not once. As I began to train, I started to notice the subtle movement of the tide—something that I had never spotted while walking, phone in hand, checking messages and chatting with mates. I saw how the birds circled at different times of day depending on how much food had been left on the beach by the tourists. I watched the shape and color of the sea shift and mottle according to what was happening in the sky above.

As autumn slowly turned to winter and the clocks changed, I learned what the seafront looked like at dusk and then in the dark. I started to cherish the sight of the sea at night and, with it, the magical feeling of having my eyes open but seeing only darkness, as if I could run off the edge of the world. I began to recognize the chandeliers and the fanciest paintings on the walls of the largest homes in the smartest crescents on the seafront. I was soon able to identify the party flats in the blocks rising above it, smiling to myself at the colored lights flashing within. I watched surfers dance on waves at dusk and ran for four miles watching a murmuration of starlings.

I learned about the Undercliff Walk, a wide esplanade cut into the chalky cliffs, running from Brighton Marina to Saltdean in the east. I would run along it, basking in the glare of the winter sun, then turn and make my way back along the top of the cliffs, feeling a few steps from flying. I would watch the Palace Pier twinkling at dusk as the lights came on, and see the West Pier seeming to bob up and down with my movement, like a regal spider in the bath.

On New Year's Day, I ran for a mile behind two emaciated, shivering Goths who hugged and huddled against each other. When I caught up with and then passed them, I wanted to embrace them both. As January took flight, I watched teams of workmen repaint the pale green Victorian railings along the front, taking a few each day, slowly making progress. Each morning I would say hello and congratulate them on getting a little farther.

When I needed to add miles to my runs, I would shimmy down narrow streets lined with fishermen's cottages and parks I'd never seen. I discovered little Tudor-style cottages and pockets of midcentury design tucked away from the endless wedding-cake prettiness of the creamy Regency seafront.

I felt myself become part of my new city as it became part

of me. I ran along the pier early one February morning, look-ing up to see a seagull hovering above, searching for doughnuts to grab. I dropped my gaze to see the sea raging beneath the wooden slats of the pier. Running between gull and water, I had never felt happier or more like I belonged. I started to under-stand the rhythm of the weird mists that appeared over the sea but never seemed to make it to land. In turn, I myself became part of the view: a runner whizzing past the tourists who daw-dled by shops filled with flip-flops and ornaments made from shells. As I enjoyed the landscape of my new city, I was also absorbed into it. Like the laces pulling the two sides of my run-ning shoes together, running was meshing me and my home closer together.

It didn't feel as if I was falling back in love with running; it felt as if I was falling deeply in love with Brighton. For the first time in my life, I had chosen a city, rather than letting my job or my father's military postings dictate where I called home. And now it was up to me to become a part of it, let it truly become part of my identity. My hair was salty with sea spray wherever I was. And I spent so much time with my legs still moving beneath me that I barely noticed I was running. Running became my meditation. Not having yet reached a point where the runs were pushing me to the point of breaking, I was able to enjoy them, thinking about the end goal and basking in the process and my surroundings.

Just as I was enjoying the gifts of running more than ever, Julia was struggling with the enormity of what she had taken on. Sadness continued to wash over her, and with it the brutal confusion of grieving for someone who had died too young.

As our marathon training ramped up, I noticed a shift in her attitude. She was preparing the ground not for victory but for potential failure. She suffered an injury in her coccyx—a nasty sprain—that caused her a huge amount of pain. She became scared to run. Her confidence stalled, then eroded. She worried about not spending enough time with her son, she worried about the amount of money we'd committed to raise, she worried about letting anyone down.

Watching her, I remembered the cast-iron belief I'd once had that I could never run a marathon. I remembered my father's calm, consistent confidence in me and how a particularly bad run had felt at times like a sort of defiance against him. I recalled with crystal clarity: I didn't doubt that I might not make it; I knew I couldn't. Now I knew I could, and I knew she could, but I didn't know how to convince her.

"But you're so much fitter than me," Julia would say.

"Only because I did the training," I replied.

"But you're a natural runner," she'd say.

"No, I am not! Have you seen my boobs? I was not born a runner. I became one."

I tried everything I could think of to reignite her self-belief—joking, pushing, ignoring, cajoling, recruiting mutual friends—but there was no convincing her. She firmly believed it was not possible.

One time we threw a trivia-night fund raiser at a bar, and I heard Julia's husband reassuring her that it didn't matter if she didn't make it. I felt despair. How dare he undermine her hard work? How dare he undermine *my* hard work? I felt like he was deliberately fueling her self-doubt. I was furious. (It was only years later, when someone said the same to me, that I understood it came from a place of unconditional love.)

As marathon day approached, Julia and I locked in a battle of wills: She became ever more convinced that she couldn't do it, and I remained sure that she could. It was as if we were determined to prove each other wrong. She was even painfully embarrassed to run in front of me, despite being strong and significantly leaner than ever before.

At one point the only thing that seemed to be impelling us both was the fact that we were raising significantly more money than we had dared to hope. We asked everyone we knew and everyone they knew for help. It was crucial that the whole endeavor had some sort of tangible result. We started compulsively checking our fund-raising site to see how the donations were totting up.

We auctioned film and TV memorabilia that we'd managed to beg, steal, and borrow. Julia arranged a sellout night of live comedy as well as the aforementioned trivia night. I wrote about our project in a national magazine, and we charted our progress online. Entire families were involved, whole friend groups. A community grew. I hoped that Julia felt the swell of goodwill toward us when she doubted herself in the dead of night, because it was certainly there; at times it was all that kept me going as I tried to maintain high spirits and confidence. Our charity was thrilled and gave us two tickets for supporters to sit with the press and VIPs at the finish line. Julia decided that she wanted her husband and friends along the course, so the tickets were sent to my delighted father. No standing on the sidelines in the rain for my parents this year.

As training progressed, the weather flip-flopped insanely between the temperatures of midwinter and midsummer. It was so hot during my seventeen-mile slog in Brighton that I ran into the sea. It was the closest I have ever come to heatstroke—the white chalk of the cliffs glowing under the beam of the sun. I dreamed of water, imagined it oozing from the ground. My tongue seemed to be growing inside my mouth like that of a dog stuck in a hot car. I waded ankle-deep into the sea, wishing I could drink it. I looked around. There were women in bikinis on the beach. It was March. I took off my running top and dipped it in the icy water. I wrung it out and put it back on. The fabric stuck to my skin, cooling me down with reassuring speed. I would make it, we would make it.

Slowly, slowly, slowly, we became fitter. On the weekend before the race, a dear friend had her bachelorette party in Dorset. I attended without touching a drop of alcohol and still had the time of my life. My confidence in my body had returned, as had my enjoyment of food and its disassociation from guilt and shame. Once more I was proud to be able to *do* rather than to watch. I spent the entire afternoon exploring the tidal pools, leaping happily from rocks into the sea like a chirpy little mountain goat. Julia texted me a couple of times, terrified that I would hurt myself and be unable to run. What she didn't know was that even if the rocks of Dorset's Jurassic coastline had smashed both of my legs to smithereens, she would not have tackled that marathon alone. I was ready.

It was not until a few days later, when we went to the London Marathon Expo in Docklands, that Julia allowed herself to believe she might make the finish line. Held at the enormous and terrifying ExCel conference center, the Expo is a three-day event where competitors collect their numbers, their running chips, and final information regarding the event. They are bombarded by corporate stands and loud vendors who hawk every conceivable type of event, outfit, shoe, power food, and accessory. The Expo is simultaneously reassuring and leg-numbingly scary. You are confronted with a world of running otherwise limited to magazines, TV footage, or word of mouth: It is a runner's mecca. It's comforting to meet other runners and discover that they are people just like you. They are dads with kids, grannies with family, friends supporting friends, and large charity groups egging one another on. Among them are many who, like Julia, are undertaking the challenge not for bravado-instilling bucket-list reasons but for emotional ones. They are making a tribute; they are offering up their suffering to help others who have suffered worse.

At the hall's entry was a large white wall steadily filling with scribbled-on messages and dedications. Julia wrote a small note to Jerome, and I signed a note next to it in support of her. As we stepped back and looked at our tiny handwriting, almost lost in the sea of others' jottings, I put my hand out and held hers. We were going to do this. We were part of something bigger than us. And we would see it through to the end.

On the morning of the event, I woke up as sick with nerves as I had three years before. This time the nerves were not about whether I could get myself round the course (which was feeling like less of a certainty) but about whether I could get Julia round it. While her anxieties had ebbed a little—and her sense of humor was doing its best to mask them—the importance of her finishing had grown with each passing day. For Jerome, for those who had helped us with the fund-raising, for those at the Royal Marsden Hospital who would be helped by the money, and for our eternally patient loved ones. We had to do them all proud.

We met at Blackheath station, where Julia presented me with a huge HEMMO badge to sew on the front of my running top.

Many close friends had used the nickname since I was in my twenties. With the advent of Twitter (and my use of "@hemmo" as my handle) and my renewed enthusiasm for running, it had become more than a nickname. It was a persona, a sportsman's moniker, a superhero identity. I was Hemmo when I was at my most "me," and Julia knew that.

As at the start of all public races, there was little space for dignity, so I whipped out the needle and thread I'd brought along and stitched the badge onto my top before asking Julia to create a temporary tent with the baggy old hoodie I was wearing and I whipped my top on beneath it. Once in Greenwich Park, we checked our bags at the luggage trucks, and I watched the dismay flicker across Julia's face as she realized that we had to surrender our valuables to a total stranger.

We took our positions in the penultimate enclosure and waited for the start to be announced. All around us, the hubbub of runners, costumes, supporters, and the incessant PA system playing "inspiring" eighties music created a carnival. We surrendered and joined in, whooping and clapping. The countdown began, and the crowd burst into cheers. We were off. It took a good ten minutes to cross the starting line, going at barely more than a shuffle, but as we did, Julia shrieked, "We're running the bloody London Marathon!"

"We so are! We so bloody are!" I shrieked back.

As with all big races, there are a few minutes, maybe half an hour, when you run along, almost in a trance, semi-hypnotized by the unfamiliar sound of hundreds of other runners. The thud of running shoes, the whispers of breath, the feeling that you can't stop because you're moving as a pack and no one's getting left behind. I tried not to talk for a bit, hoping that Julia would absorb and enjoy the moment, letting confidence and pride seep in. We ran in silence before I cracked and let out the first of many hollers on seeing our friends Jon and Dave standing at the side of the road. Arms crossed, feet hip-width apart and eyes glazed, they had led the charge with teasing us about training over the last few months. Now they were there for us. Up early on a Sunday, as steadfast and honorable as I'd always suspected they were.

"GUYS!" I shouted, and their blank gazes broke into goofy grins and big lollopy waves. They shouted back and carried on cheering until we were long gone. I felt a lump in my throat: The first of many supporters had seen us making a go of it. Julia was glowing at the sheer exhilaration of being cheered in the streets.

The bands, the crowds, the children with their little pots of jelly beans: The atmosphere alone kept us going for the first few miles. Soon we were approaching Tower Bridge and the halfway mark. The heat was rising. The unpredictable weather had settled on "blazing summer day." I kept encouraging Julia to drink water and was barely without a bottle in my hand myself. It seemed prudent to walk for a portion of each mile, rather than to overheat before the end. Even the spectators looked roasting.

As we got to the bridge, I told Julia we should run. "You don't want to wake up tomorrow and say that you walked over Tower Bridge," I insisted.

"I'm not sure how well I'm doing," she replied.

"It doesn't matter! We're not going for a time! It's an experience you'll never repeat!"

"I don't know . . ."

"Please! For me! Why don't you run ahead a bit, and I'll take a picture!"

Julia was persuaded. The photograph I took is one of my favorites, with her looking over one shoulder and an image of

Jerome on the back of her T-shirt. We held hands aloft over the second half of the bridge, screaming with delight.

Not long after the halfway mark, the heat and the exhaustion started to take their toll. The sunshine was merciless; there didn't seem to be enough water on earth to keep us cool. I tried pouring it down the back of Julia's neck, and we took turns squealing through the showers at the side of the road.

When you're running, heat doesn't just make you feel hot— it chips away at your reality, slowly but surely. It makes your feet feel as if you're wearing someone else's oversize shoes. It makes your tongue feel as if you have woken up with the worst hangover of your life. Worst of all, it can confuse you. Distances start to lose perspective, limbs feel heavy, and words begin to jumble.

During a marathon, perfectly normal, reasonable physiological responses to heat suddenly feel like emotional Armageddon. While I knew that the third quarter of a marathon felt like hell, I knew that it didn't last forever. Julia did not. To watch her slump was heartrending. The longer a run is, the less it becomes about running. The challenge is dealing with the waves of emotion, keeping the mind from collapsing. As anyone who has started from scratch knows, emotions carried around for several miles can feel heavier than hell itself.

Throughout training, I'd seen Julia find threads of confidence and hope in running, to retrieve her pre-baby body and feel stronger than ever. That Julia was fading in front of me. Her shoulders slumped, her feet struggled to lift in the heat, and the face that had earlier been alert and positive, looking out at the spectacle, was now downcast. Where she was waving brightly at strangers, she was now avoiding their gaze. Where our shared sense of humor had seemed so infallible, my cajoling now met her ears as goading.

Our pace slowed and our faces reddened. I felt utterly helpless, seeing Julia losing every last scrap of self-belief. To say that she was convinced we wouldn't finish would be an understatement—she seemed almost affronted that I had the temerity to suggest otherwise. Every "You *can* do this, I know you can!" was met with an even sharper "No, I *can't*! Why don't you *understand*?"

Ever grateful that I had been down this dark road and slugged it out with my dad's support, I tried to let her protestations ride over me. They still stung, as the exhaustion was far from easy for me. I channeled my father's unwavering faith and kept talking, kept encouraging, kept distracting. At times I was so hot that I wasn't sure if I was hallucinating. Words upon words came spilling out of my mouth until I no longer really knew what my latest profundity was. A quote from Eleanor Roosevelt? Or perhaps something from *Dawson's Creek*. No matter, as long as we kept going forward, forward.

Toward the end of the race, I felt Julia was truly at her darkest, almost physically exfoliating herself of layer upon layer of grief. Her emotional pain was mirrored by considerable physical pain. I encouraged her to let it all out. If she could cry here on the street, maybe there would be less sadness when she got home, I reasoned.

Slowly, eventually, we turned onto the Embankment and saw more familiar faces. I had been talking up the "last-mile high" since we started. Julia was struggling. For months I had been telling her that this moment would be worth it. And then we were there. But even as we turned onto the Mall, she was expressing doubt that she would make it.

"I can carry you from here!" I yelled, sure that her spirits would rally soon.

"Oh my God, oh my God."

"What?"

"I can see the finish line!" A huge grin cracked her face. Finally, she knew she could do it.

As we ran toward the finish line, I took her hand. We heard people shouting our names. I couldn't work out where the voices were coming from. As we approached the gallery of press seats at the finish line, I saw my parents: my father in his seat, grinning and waving wildly, and my mother, shrieking and clambering down from the seats and onto the side of the track. She scuttled toward us as the sound of her voice cut over the music and cheering. "GO GO GO ALEX AND JULIA YOU ARE THE BEST YOU MUST KEEP GOING EVERYONE IS SO PROUD OF YOU, YOU HAVE NO IDEA HOW PROUD WE ALL ARE AND NOW IT IS THE FINISH JUST ENJOY IT I HAVE BEEN SITTING HERE ALL DAY AND SEEN SO MUCH BORING SPORT AND NOW YOU ARE FINALLY HERE OH THANK GOD GO GO GO GO ALEX AND JULIA . . ."

She was off the seating area and running alongside us, my father behind her in the stands, taking photographs. She continued to run along with us, screaming, until we ran our final steps. We crossed the finish line, grinning, crying, holding hands.

We had done it.

We collected our medals and bags and headed to the crowd of friends and family waiting for us with hugs, food, and congratulations. A friend's little boy paraded around wearing my medal, convinced he had won the marathon. My mother cried and stroked my hair. Julia hugged her son, who was wearing her medal.

We had done it.

* * *

I lay facedown on a massage table the next day, staring at the masseuse's feet: a moment of stillness after the shouting, heaving, and weeping of the previous day. I watched the feet shuffle gently out of view and realized that something had shifted in me. While you, and only you, can move your legs from start to finish, no one runs a marathon alone. Though I had supported Julia, I had received great support myself. My friends and family knew how hard I'd found it, and they had been wonderful. But what I had really learned was that running could no longer be about me and my personal goals. To go that far, to feel that pain, to endure that depth of despair, it had to be about more than my own self-worth; it had to have a purpose beyond me. I couldn't continue running around in circles.

As soon as I could, I opened my laptop and bought places for several races over the course of the next year: the Royal Parks Foundation Half Marathon; the White Night Half Marathon; the Brighton Half Marathon; and the Brighton Marathon.

I had to reach further. I had to reach beyond myself.

8

A Runner for Life?

Methinks that the moment my legs begin to move,
my thoughts begin to flow . . .

—Henry David Thoreau

My ambition in the first few days after my second London Marathon was at an all-time high. Without Julia to coax, I was sure that I would be able to touch the outer limits of my ability. I had given myself two months to rest before training for two half marathons, which were to take place in October and February, followed by the Brighton Marathon in April. These would be my real runs, my masterworks! I would discover the truth about myself on those courses and then head to Edinburgh to conquer Arthur's Seat. And I had my heart set on securing a place in the Women's Marathon in San Francisco, a city I'd long fantasized about, that October.

A week later, I was on holiday in Rome, hobbling around the Forum on still-tired feet and burying my face in pasta at every available opportunity. Six months later, the fire I once had in my belly seemed to have dimmed. Running was less a series of exciting adventures than a habit. It had slotted into the routine of my life, a pleasant enough pastime, though I had the nagging feeling that I was putting a little more into it than I was getting out. Still, it had been a sunny summer, and I remained uninjured, so I had stuck with the program, more or less, and looked forward to the gentle goal of the Royal Parks Half Marathon in October.

That September I went to the cinema in London to watch Ryan Gosling in *Drive*. It's great, I recommend it, but remember: I saw him first. It is hard for me to be distracted when I am in the beam of The Gosling, so when my phone vibrated as I entered the cinema, I answered only because it was my sister's due date for her first baby and I could see that it was my mother calling. Instead of being told that my sister had been admitted to the hospital, I was told that her husband, a healthy, active thirty-five-year-old, was lying in a ward. His heart rate was dangerously elevated, and no one knew why. My mother told me to go into the film, as there was nothing any of us could do until he had seen a specialist, but she asked me to keep my mobile on in case my sister needed me. I entered the cinema in a semi-trance, my blood icy in my veins.

I sat with my phone in my hand, hypnotized by Gosling, yet aware of a constant ticker tape of anxiety scrolling across my mind. What was happening in the hospital a few miles away? I didn't understand. I texted my father throughout the film to see if there were any updates: no news yet. I left the cinema and telephoned St. George's Hospital. I knew that the situation was not good when I was put directly through to my sister within seconds. She was in tears and asked me to come immediately.

What followed was one of the most extraordinary forty-eight hours of all of our lives. I met my sister, headed home, made her some toast and tea, helped her in and out of the bath, and put her to bed. There was no sign of their baby; nor was there any sign of her husband, who remained attached to myriad mysterious hospital wires. The next morning I accompanied my sister to the midwife, then to the hospital to see her husband. I looked away when he told her that he was going into emergency heart surgery in a matter of hours. I held my breath when I heard him ask the surgeon what the alternative was. I did not breathe out when the reply came. "There is none. Your condition is very rare, and fatal if untreated."

My sister was advised to go home and rest while the surgery took place, and that the procedure would take two to three hours. Resting was easier said than done; it took us ten minutes to get her upstairs, wracked as she was with sobs of despair. I went downstairs and made three dishes of lasagna, wishing I had my running shoes. I was still wearing the same outfit I'd left for the cinema in the previous day.

Four hours later, we had heard nothing. My sister sat at the kitchen table and pressed redial for thirty minutes. Eventually, we were told we could go and visit. Amazingly, her husband was fine, his condition cured entirely by pioneering keyhole surgery. The next morning my sister went into labor and had a beautiful, healthy baby boy: Louis.

A week later, I ran the Royal Parks Foundation Half Marathon in London, as planned. There had been a point when I wondered if I'd be able to make it, but in the end it seemed like the only sensible thing to do. The previous week had been spent in a flurry of e-mails and phone calls, recounting the story of the extraordinary turn of events again and again. I visited the family, I visited my friends, I visited everyone I loved and could reach. I wanted to hug them all. I told the story until it was ragged, worn away by retelling, until it started to seem like a plotline from a soap opera I was summarizing for a stranger. It was almost as if it hadn't happened to me.

I was nervous the morning of the run, as I always am when I go to a big public event alone. Had I forgotten something? Who would get me home to Brighton if I fell? Would this finally be the race where I wet myself in front of a crowd of onlookers? The usual worries. Race aside, I felt happy and relaxed after a week in the company of those I loved, grappling with the dramatic but ultimately joyous news.

As I crossed the starting line, I felt a little emotional at how beautiful London looked that day. It had been a bizarre year for weather, and while there had been rain that morning, the autumn sky was now gorgeously crisp, and the leaves in Hyde Park were exquisite. I felt a little lump in my throat as we left the park and headed out along the Mall, then down along the river. We crossed at Waterloo Bridge and began to run back. That was when it happened. The tears.

Initially, I thought it was a tiny eye leak, the kind you might get at a moving political speech or a great novel. You know, if you've had the right amount of whiskey and some good company. A moment in passing. But the tears that initially could be mistaken for eyes streaming from the cold soon turned into heaving sobs.

The first one appeared as a half-gulp, half-yelp. The second one was an identifiable gasp. Five miles into a half marathon, I was off—proper full-blown crying. I didn't know what was wrong with me: I wasn't sad; in fact, I was very happy. The news was all good, wasn't it? Yet it seemed that after almost a fortnight of coping, my body and mind had decided to unburden at mile five, in the anonymity of the crowd. Only I wasn't anonymous; I was wearing a top bearing my nickname, HEMMO, in eight-inch letters. By the time I realized this, a thousand feelings per second had started to course through me, as if I were some sort of magical emotion kaleidoscope. Every other second came a fresh sensation I hadn't let myself feel in front of my sister, the surgeons, or anyone in the hospital. It was a tidal wave of tears.

Before I knew it, my sobs were almost uncontrollable, to the point where the rhythm of my feet on the pavement had become the only thing stopping me from losing it altogether. I don't know how I managed to keep running, yet it was all that I could do. The memories of the previous ten days flashed before me: my hand round my mobile in that dark cinema as I waited for news; my sister's hand as she signed the consent form for her husband's surgery; my brother-in-law's hand as he stroked her bump. The smell of the antiseptic in the hospital, the smell of the food I made while my sister slept, the smell of my newborn nephew's head. Flashes of the conversations I had been having for days on end, until they lost all meaning to me, flooded back into my consciousness: "What, he could have died?" "What, the baby was born the next day?" "What, you're still going to run at the weekend?"

Of course I still ran; it was a habit. The date was in the diary, immovable. As I now realized, it was only through running that

I was able to process how traumatic those few days had been. Except the spectators along the route that day didn't know the reason for my sobs. They just saw a runner in distress and cheered me on. Which, if I am honest, only made things worse. Because with every step, my heart seemed to be swelling—expanding to make room for this newly realized love I felt for my brother-in-law, my new nephew, and the friends who had supported us all. There wasn't space to love the sweet faces of the children who had come out to support a dad or a sibling and found themselves cheering me along too. Was there? So their kindness was converted into more grinning tears as I gulped and tried to smile back and explain: "Oh no, don't worry, I'm fine! It's just that . . ." and I was past them.

"WELL DONE, HEMMO," they shrieked at my back. And that just made me cry more.

Calm down, you're embarrassing yourself now, you need to get your heart rate down if you're going to carry on, I told myself, which only prompted further tears at the very thought of hearts. *Oh, hearts! Hearts are so amazing!* Once again I was lost in the wonder of life itself.

I don't remember the last couple of miles, until I reached the final straight. I saw the finish line and felt a strength I didn't know I had. Admittedly I had not run exceptionally fast, given my busy schedule of weeping, but I felt more powerful than ever. My brother-in-law had survived. My sister had survived. We had all survived. So I sprinted. I felt myself speed up until I could see that I was overtaking the people around me. I left them behind, running faster than I ever had. Slowly, I felt my face begin to tingle, then my hands. As I came within meters of the finish line, I wondered if I was going to make it at all. I did, straight into the arms of a St. John Ambulance worker who had seen me coming. He tilted my head forward over my knees to steady my breathing, which was now hysterical. I thanked him through my weird gulpy gasps, and with relief I took the water he gave me. Moments later, my brother appeared and bought me a sausage in a bun. It was the best sausage in a bun I have ever known, and they are *always* good. On the train home, I e-mailed my girlfriends the story, expecting to be told I was quite mad. But they understood. They understood it all.

That day in October was the day that taught me so much about why I run. It wasn't a habit, it was a necessity: the essential realization that I can carry on when I am sure I am about to die; that to survive, I just have to keep going, keeping the faith that I could leave the house almost trembling with trepidation about what lay ahead, and if I could keep myself going, a few minutes, a few lampposts, a few blocks at a time, I would be improving not just my running but how I managed my life.

Slowly, as the seasons changed, so did my legs and my lungs. I clung to my realization that those moments of anger or desolation at desperate points of a lengthy run were basic physiological reactions to the situation. I told myself that if I could accept what they were, then I could learn to conquer them, and then I might begin to believe that anything was possible. I ran during the Christmas break and even went for a New Year's Day run after a particularly gleeful New Year's Eve party at a friend's house on the seafront. Queasy from champagne and dodgy cocktails, I left the house on legs like Bambi's, frail but determined to start the year undefeated. I tottered along the seafront only to be greeted by the entire house party from the night before, cheering and whooping from the doorstep as I passed. Walkers, only their eyes visible amidst hats and scarves, turned to stare, curious about this lunatic woman shrieking, "I might yet spew!" at a Regency villa. By the time I was home, my hangover was gone, replaced with a more honest tiredness and a renewed sense of my own resilience.

Sixteen weeks later was my birthday, the weekend of the Brighton Half Marathon. After applying two years earlier and not making it due to food poisoning, then attempting it the year before with Julia and pulling out within a mile on account of further illness, I was worried that I was blighted by my guts when it came to running in my hometown. This year I was the fittest I had ever been. I knew a half marathon was not an unreasonable race, and I had friends and family, including my now adorably rotund nephew, Louis, coming down to cheer me on and enjoy a big birthday lunch afterward. I wanted it to be a happy race. I decided it would be a happy race. Perhaps because of that, it was. It was the happiest race I have ever run.

The moods caused by running are part of a delicate and mysterious alchemy. I will never forget the boiling rage I experienced on my way through Hyde Park a few years before. It was a bitterly cold January day, a training run for my first London Marathon. I was aiming for eleven miles, the farthest I had ever run in my life and farther than I could have imagined I'd be able to go only three months previously.

The sky was so crisp that the world looked like it was being broadcast in high definition, and the ground underfoot was frosty in places. I had my hands balled into fists within my running gloves and my phone in the pocket of my thermal running tights. I had managed about five or six miles—which was by then an average midweek run—without too much of a problem. About twenty minutes later, I started to feel tragically tired. My fingers were losing sensation in the cold, my face was becoming brittle from bracing itself against the wind, and my thighs felt like liquid lead. I was eight miles in and sure I would have to lie on Park Lane and beg a taxi to take me home.

Then I saw them. On the north side of the park. Together. The couple holding hands. Nothing wrong with holding hands on a lovely Sunday walk, I can hear you say. But they weren't on a lovely Sunday walk. They were runners. Runners holding hands. A his-and-hers run. Matching slinky running tights, matching headbands, and fully synchronized strides. And their hands clasped between them. Who does that? And why? Who are these people who are so inseparable that they need physical contact *maintained* while running? My rage was as pure and brilliant as the snow sitting on the duck pond.

Then there have been the times when I have been frustrated beyond comprehension by dawdling shoppers crossing a road, or desperate with loneliness at the farthest point from home, or almost delirious with joy on realizing that I have run for three miles with almost no recollection of it. It is these moments of meditative blankness, followed by piercing clarity: That is the feeling you're chasing on the best runs.

For this half marathon I held that feeling, as solid and spar-kling as a diamond, for almost the entire run. The weather, the sky, and the sea were exquisite. I felt as if every breath I took in went directly to my muscles, my organs, my spirit. I have never felt more like a runner. I don't know why. Perhaps it was because instead of running filled with fear, I wanted to run as quickly as possible so I could see my friends and family. I was so happy that they had come down to support me on home turf, and so excited to see my nephew, little Louis. I honestly believed I was running directly into their arms that day. I felt golden, untouchable.

After plumbing the emotional depths in the autumn, I felt that my suspicions had been proved right—you had to keep at it. I had to decide that it would get better, just as I'd had to decide that I could become a runner. In both instances, the training had been secondary to the mental resilience required. Now, as I sat at that lunch table, surrounded by the debris of gift wrapping and empty plates, with my most beloved around me, I was reaping the rewards. I hadn't trained only my legs; I was learning to train my brain. They were finally working together instead of against each other. How could I make it last?

Six weeks later, I was on another training run, this time a ten-mile race around Salisbury, near my parents' house. We started at a local sports center in the north of the city and headed up through breathtaking scenery along the Wye Valley. As we chased the river alongside fields full of frolicking spring-time lambs and trees full of playful birds, I felt a rush at the extraordinary views that my running afforded me. I realized that I was going at almost exactly the same pace as two men ahead of me. They looked strong and fit. They had the physique of runners who usually left me far behind within the first half mile of an event.

One of the greatest joys of running is how unexpected body shapes manage to run at speeds and distances that seem to bear no relation to their size. I have been overtaken by several women at least twenty years older than I am on the Brighton seafront (including one, my nemesis, who seems to manage it once a month). Similarly, I have overtaken gobsmackingly athletic-looking women who are clearly younger but haven't put in the same number of miles. Best of all is overtaking the men. The first time I did this was on one of my first Brighton runs, when I plodded along for about a mile behind a man whose

T-shirt declared him "born to run" and whose smell betrayed him as a fan of Axe body spray instead of a shower.

I tried for about eight minutes to overtake him, knowing that if I were going to succeed, I would have to save enough energy to stay ahead of him, as the path was long and straight—there was little room for turning off in shame. After running alongside him for about thirty seconds, I managed it. The man might have been seriously ill in his recent past. He might have had all sorts of problems I will never know about. But he was a man, and he was about my age, so it felt like a huge victory to be able to pass him.

That day in Salisbury I decided to try it again. I was sure that once we had passed the brow of that hill, I would be able to make it. I steadied myself, and then, as we descended, I tried to catch them. As I got closer, I realized that the man on the right was describing the view to his companion. I assumed that it was some sort of concentration exercise; I had been known to count sheep or lampposts. I slowed, running in sync with them for a bit. I observed that the companion was barely replying, using grunts rather than words. Who was this rude man? Able-bodied, running with a mate, and yet entirely ignoring him. I gave myself a little push and tried to get close enough to read the text on his running vest. Whichever snooty running club he was a member of would be one I'd be sure to give a miss. Having accelerated a little, I decided to go for it and overtake them. I'd had enough of the strange dynamic; it was only going to irritate me if I carried on so close to them. As I drew up, I glanced to my right, poised to give the surly runner a sneer, to let him know what I thought of the way he was treating his companion.

He never would have seen me, because he barely had a face. At first I thought that the sunlight was dappling shadow across his features. But no, he really did have only half a face. It was as I glanced at him, trying my best not to stumble in shock, that I saw the text on his vest was that of an army regiment. I understood that he was probably a veteran of the war in Afghanistan. And his injuries were profound. Where once there would have been eyes, there were only smooth scars. Likewise one of his ears. All of this above a body in perfect working condition. I swallowed and ran on, stunned by what I'd seen and ashamed of my knee-jerk assumptions.

Those mornings when I hadn't felt like going on runs, when I felt the ghost of a hangover, when I chose to watch dross on TV instead of doing my stretches, seemed ridiculous now. Here was a man half destroyed by war, choosing to push his body to the limit, while his mate described the scenery. I reached the finish line transfixed by thoughts of the opportunities I had and how little I made of them. It was a perfect boost to my training for the Brighton Marathon the following month, which I was more committed to than ever.

9

Runner's High

*Stadiums are for spectators. We runners have nature and
that is much better.*

—Juha Väätäinen

*I*f my first marathon had been about seeing whether I could
do it, and my second had been about helping a friend make
a dream come true, my third was about finding out what I was
capable of. I wanted to know how far I could push myself, how
fast I could go over a marathon distance, and how successfully
I could harness my emotions.

There was nowhere to hide. I was running a marathon in my
hometown, injury-free. No excuses. Before I had busied myself
by attaching emotive monikers to my endeavors, as if they were
lost episodes of *Friends:* The Lonely One, The Enraged One,
The Sobbing One. This time I would approach the project like a
machine. A marathon machine.

Things went better than I could have hoped. I trained hard
throughout the spring. I was disciplined about losing a bit of
weight, so there was less Hemmo to carry along the course. I did

my stretches, and I worked hard with a trainer—the unfailingly patient Adam, whom I had been seeing for eighteen months. When I'd committed to running the London Marathon with Julia, I had found a trainer I could work with occasionally to strengthen the muscles from which I needed the most support when running. The memories of my injury—and the tedium of the physio exercises—I had endured the first time round convinced me that parting with what felt like an extravagant sum was worth it. Adam, a keen triathlete and well-qualified trainer, was my age and knew I was interested in the science of what was going on in my body and had little interest in being "beasted," military fitness–style. His encouragement and practical approach to my physiology (and emotional roller coaster) has worked wonders. I remained uninjured.

Gradually, I relearned the lesson that I ran to improve my life; I didn't improve my life in order to run. I ate better than I ever had, forcing myself to love oat smoothies under the tutelage of the former flatmate whose North London runs I had envied all those years ago. I took part in local park runs every Saturday and felt buoyed by the communal effort; I focused on fund-raising to make sure that for every aching muscle I suffered, I was reminded that there were others in greater pain. I took resting seriously for the first time in my life and didn't regret saying no to the odd night out. I was sleeping better than I ever had. I relished the admiration that the garbagemen expressed when I lifted almost the same amount they did with ease. The routine propelled me forward, freeing me to be more creative in other areas. I ran along the seafront, I ran across the Downs, I ran myself happy. I was ready for my third marathon.

Until tonsillitis. At first I thought I was tired. Then I thought

I had a sore throat. Next came the shivers. Two days before the marathon, I showed my throat to a friend who took one look, shrieked, and announced, "You look as if you have babies' anuses down there." It was a low point.

The next day I tried calling my doctor to see if I could get an appointment. She said she would leave me a prescription at the pharmacy, which I duly collected. Tonsillitis it was. Though my hopes of running a strong marathon had faded, I wanted to know if I could at least make the starting line. I didn't care if I ran a slow time, but I wanted to take part in the event for which I had been training six months, the one that ran straight past my front door. My only concern was lasting damage. In endurance running, there is a fine line between gritty courage and downright dumb-ass bravado. I preferred to stay on the alive side of that line. I tried calling my doctor to ask whether I should run, but the office was closed.

I put out a plea on Twitter in case there were any doctors online who could help. I received a barrage of answers about people having heart attacks and inflamed brains, along with plenty of other horror stories that only the Internet could provide. There was one useful tweet: A friend pointed me in the direction of Tim Weeks, a trainer who offered to call me. Moments later, I was talking through my symptoms with him, as he is a hugely experienced runner and trainer, and his wife is a doctor.

"I don't mind it if it's hard; it's going to be hard anyway. I just don't want to be a fool and damage myself in the long term," I explained.

"You won't do that with tonsillitis," he reassured me.

"Are you sure? I have a lot of friends telling me not to run. . . ."

"I am sure. But if you start, you should do so having accepted that you might not finish."

"That's the opposite of everything you're told about setting out for a marathon!"

"Yes, but you clearly have tonsillitis. You are in a weakened state. Just keep your chest covered for as long as you can when you start. And don't expect too much of yourself."

The next morning I set off for Brighton's Preston Park with a long-sleeved top on and three scarves in my bag. Handing over my bag left me with a slightly limbless sensation, as if I were missing more than just a few possessions. It was me and my body at the start line, ready for another expedition into the unknown.

The first half of the marathon was a breeze. I kept covered up for well over an hour and received a steady trickle of texts from friends, family, and the lovely Tim Weeks. As we hit the seafront, I saw Julia, waving like a maniac at me on the side of the road, and soon we had covered the distance of a half marathon. I received a text from my brother to say that he had just completed the Paris Marathon. I ran past the square where I lived; I saw more friends and even my neighbors out on the street, shouting and cheering. Then, at around mile twenty, I abruptly felt as if someone had pulled a stopper out of me. I had never eaten or trained better for a race in my life, but I felt utterly bloodless. It was something I had never felt, even in the extremes of exhaustion. This wasn't just tiredness; it was a bodily refusal to engage. I stopped at the next water station and took two drinks, which I sipped while walking slowly on the side of the road. I gave myself a pep talk and decided to continue.

As with the London Marathon, a significant chunk of the second half of the course was in a large industrial space. It went past the Shoreham power station and a powerfully depressing sewage works. My brain was looping, telling me off for not having trained properly, for being weak, for not having the mental rigor to achieve my goals. *You're just tired, you have an illness,* I kept trying to tell myself, only to have my brain reply louder each time, reminding me of my inadequacies. We plodded past iron gates and concrete wastelands while this hideous internal dialogue continued to torment me: *You're not good enough. It's not even that you're not good enough, it's that you can't get any better. You're just not good.*

Eventually, I couldn't take it anymore and slowed to a walk, a heaving sob in the well of my stomach.

"You can't stop," said a voice behind me.

I didn't turn around. I wasn't in the mood.

"Seriously, you can't stop," the voice repeated. "You're the only thing keeping me going."

I turned and saw a bloke about my age, running a couple of feet behind me. I raised my eyebrows at him. Well, I tried to. Even my eyebrows were exhausted.

"Honestly, I've been watching your feet and trying to keep mine in time with yours. It's the only thing that has kept me running since we were back there." He waved a hand dismissively, suggesting that his opinion of a Sunday spent touring a sewage farm was as favorable as mine. "If you stop running, I will have to stop running, and I don't want to let my friend down."

"Well, where is your friend?" I asked, dragging myself back into a run.

"He's gone ahead. But we were running this together for his mum."

"Oh no. Is she okay?"

"No, she died of cancer a few months ago. I said I would run the marathon with him to raise money for the hospice where she was."

"Oh." I felt stilled. Perhaps my woes weren't quite that bad. "I'm sorry."

"It's okay, but really, you have to keep me running. I can't flake out now."

"Yes, you're right, we really do have to keep running, don't we?"

"Yes."

"Deal," I said. "I'm Alex."

"And I'm Nick. Nice to meet you." We shook hands.

"I won't leave you until this is done," I said.

Run we did. For the last five miles of that marathon, we plodded along together, not fast but not walking. I promised him for miles that there were friends at a house on the seafront, waiting to cheer us. It seemed like weeks until we got back to Hove, but when we did, what a greeting! They had made bunting! They were having an actual party! I waved and pointed at Nick, yelling, "This is Nick!" until they all cheered for him too. As we approached the last mile, his supporters did the same for me, and I beamed as his girlfriend caught his eye, tearfully proud.

When we got to the finish line, nineteen minutes after the four-hour-and-thirty-minute time I had been hoping to achieve, we shared the kind of hug that you can have only with a total stranger you have shared an intense experience with. I had learned more about Nick in that last hour than I ever found out about people I'd worked with for years. I heard about his work rebuilding the *Cutty Sark,* and I told him about running past it in the London Marathon. I told him about my family, and he told me about the friend he was running to support. We had battled forward, part of that collective endeavor to convert energy to money, to aid, to solace. We were making something bigger than salt, sweat, and swollen feet. Only the two of us knew how horrible those last few miles had been, how spirit-crushing our internal mechanisms could be, and how sometimes it is only the hand of a stranger extended toward you that can get you to the very end. When we got there, it was all the sweeter for it.

"I'll rest!" I promised my friends, who were muttering darkly about me overdoing things. And rest I did. I stayed at home in my deliciously ugly compression socks, eating whatever I wanted and catching up on ridiculous television. When I was better, I spent a month going to parties wearing silly heels. I enjoyed myself doing whatever I wanted, letting routine's grip relax a little. I kept up with a few park runs and did some social runs with my sister, who was busy losing her baby weight by running around the parks and commons of South London. I enjoyed the lack of pressure, letting myself acquiesce to the fact that no matter how hard you train, chasing a time or fund-raising target need not be the focus. My acceptance and enjoyment were a delight, and running brought me unmitigated gentle pleasures for months.

Then came the e-mail. Edinburgh. I had forgotten about Edinburgh. During my post–London Marathon madness the year before, one of the more "fun" runs I had applied to was called the Speed of Light: a live running installation that would be part of the world-famous Edinburgh Arts Festival. Its aims sounded lofty—"a desire to elevate non-elite distance and endurance running to the realms of the extraordinary"— but the practicalities really bewitched me. Put together by a public art collective, the proposal was for a group of runners to wear bespoke LED suits controlled from a distance, which meant that they would change color, brightness, and the speed at which they flashed. We would run across the crags of Arthur's Seat in formation, as taught by a choreographer, at different speeds, creating an elegant cross between Tron and a host of fireflies on the hilltop. In my post-marathon flush of enthusiasm, I was determined to be a part of this event. It wasn't just childish excitement about donning a space-age suit that had fired my imagination; it was being part of a statement that running needn't always be about distance or time. That there could be beauty and validity in the act. Yes, the more I thought about it, the more I believed that *this* was the event for me.

But as time had passed, the communication from NVA, the organizers, had been very infrequent. I hadn't been convinced it would happen—my perception of the Edinburgh Festival had been tainted by that of the Fringe: a pub table of twenty-two-year-old stoners trying to find a back room for some improv. If it did happen, I thought it would be much more about spectacle than any sense of athleticism. I'd forgotten about the event and about training for it. After all, it was four months after the Brighton Marathon. Until the morning I sat in bed with my laptop, some toast and peanut butter, and a coffee, and saw the e-mail. About training.

RUNNING LIKE A GIRL

Whereas e-mails from the London Marathon usually arrive via the charity you are running for and are chatty blocks of text gearing you up for the challenge, this was a video. Of a man looking very angry on top of a hill. The man was Angus Farquhar, the organizer of the event, which was to comprise groups of runners in full-body light suits, running up and down Arthur's Seat in the dark, creating stunning visual effects for the spectators, who would be watching live on the hill. While I had been excited by the event, now I was exhausted. And terrified.

The video began with a stern talk about how hill training was different from any other form of training, that if you could run ten miles confidently on the flat, you still might struggle with the challenges that Arthur's Seat presented. "Doing a few road runs will be a complete nightmare. You simply will not be able to keep the pace up, and keeping the pace up is essential," warned Angus as the wind came straight off the sea and ruffled his hair vigorously. "If, after ten minutes, you need to walk, your whole group will have to walk, and the whole beautiful effect of this work will be destroyed."

Running as art didn't feel like it was going to be that much fun. Angus spoke sternly of the type of training needed and of how we WOULD NOT COPE if we did not complete it. "There is no magic to hill work; you just have to go out and train on hills." Fair enough, but Angus, please, a smile would not hurt. There followed an even sterner talk about footwear. We were to buy proper trail shoes. Anyone in a regular pair of running shoes was a fool, as good as taking her life into her own hands.

The camera focused again on Angus, looking increasingly livid. A final word. "I said we were on steep terrain; we are actually on the edge of a cliff, Salisbury Crags." The camera panned past Angus to show a vertical drop of nearly fifty meters. "But don't worry, we will never go within two meters of the cliff. It will be really easy to trip."

Within two meters! With wind that stiff, it didn't seem like much at all. My heart rate had been rising steadily. I forwarded the video to Adam, my trainer, with a bold "LOL!" beneath it. His response wasn't quite as chirpy; the text that pinged back almost immediately announced a change in tactics. I would have to up my running. Again. It was time to learn to run on rough terrain, and it was time to run at night. I guiltily kicked a new pair of heels under my bed and looked up some tips on hill training.

It was a full moon for my first night run on the South Downs. Adam and I had set out at ten P.M., as early as we could have done, given the late July weather. Dusk was falling as we drove out of Brighton, and by the time we set off from Devil's Dyke for Truleigh Hill, the moon was almost directly above us. While I had grown to love runs after dark along the seafront, I still gasped when we reached the top of the first hill and I looked out toward Brighton. The sea was visible, the moon reflected in it. The scene was the sort of thing a Goth teenager might have on a bedroom wall, complete with a sympathetic yet masterful wolf at one side, howling. I was wearing my headlamp from the White Night Half Marathon, and Adam was carrying a flashlight. The galloping sensation of running over chunks of chalk and flint was utterly different from the reliability of hitting tarmac or pavement. I could feel each of the muscles and bones in my feet pulling together, getting stronger and having a strange sort of fun as they tried to work out what they would hit with the next step. I felt my heart rate increase as I headed up and up, and I felt my body giggle as I juddered down a hill, using all the core body strength I had built with Adam to stop me from toppling over entirely. I got home after midnight, excited. I didn't need to be scared; I was going to become art after all!

On the night of the event, I realized that no matter how lofty my artistic ambitions had been, they could not save me from the enormity of Arthur's Seat. It was a Saturday in midsummer, and as I headed through central Edinburgh, the entire city seemed to be warming up for the mother of all parties. I paced through the streets in my nerdy little trail shoes and merino-wool running top, past bars humming with the nervous energy and lip-glossed hope of a good Saturday night. I headed out of the city and to the tiny city of marquees housing the event and equipment at the bottom of the hill. We gathered in groups and then walked out onto the hill to hear a run-through of our routines. We would be running in circles, zigzags, and other patterns across the landscape, wearing our light suits like wannabe spacemen, and holding special flashlights that lit up when shaken. Excitement bubbled through the group, and I felt a flicker of smugness at those I had passed on the way. Pah! I was going to be the one having the magical Saturday night after all.

Dusk was falling, and a TV in a corner of one of the marquees was broadcasting the final Saturday night of the Olympics as Angus gave us a pep talk about the event. He began with some characteristically stern words about how the environment up on Arthur's Seat was "very serious at night." "It can turn on you," he told us. "The terrain is rough, and the mist can come in just like that." I stifled a nervous giggle. As he continued to talk, my fear gave way to a sense of wonder. Running is a generous act, he explained, and the energy we were creating would be helping to power the light suits and the torches, rather than simply being calories expended for our own good, to hit a time goal or shift a few pounds. Our movement would be translated into light to be shared and enjoyed by others. He cracked a smile at the end. I was spellbound.

At about eleven P.M., we set out for the hill. The light suits were heavier than I had expected, covering our arms, legs, and torsos. As we began to run slowly, steadily, but always in formation, euphoria came over me. As we approached each craggy hill, I felt a thrill as I realized my legs and heart were more than strong enough to keep me constant regardless of the terrain. I had the power to go uphill and not gallop away when we headed downhill. I heard animals in the undergrowth; I heard the gasps of the audience as we burst into little star shapes of energy on the side of the hill; I heard the panting of the ten of us in my group, running in silence. A whole new world of running seemed to be opening up to me, one where goals, times, and distances were not important; just running across a landscape and feeling it underfoot was enough.

As I walked back to my hotel through the now rather tired-looking streets of Edinburgh, I tried to see myself through the eyes of those who had come to watch the event. *What sort of person does that?* they must have been thinking. It was undeniably beautiful, but also a sort of madness. I tried to see myself through the eyes of my friends and family who had been watching my progress all year. *What is she up to?* they must have been wondering. Running was no longer how I stayed fit but who I was. It was how I functioned, how I relaxed, how I processed my emotions. It was something that those who loved me, loved *about* me.

10

The Right to Run

Running gives freedom. When you run you can determine your own tempo. You can choose your own course and think whatever you want. Nobody tells you what to do.

—Nina Kuscik

Oh, how magnificent I felt as I sat on the train back from Edinburgh. While the gorgeous voluptuousness of the Cumbrian hills whizzed by, I felt as if I were part of them. My running had melded me with the landscape all over again. I stared at the cleavage of a valley, knowing what the gentle give of the turf felt like beneath my feet. My eyes softened as we passed a lake and I remembered the glassy water of the Firth of Forth as I stared out over Edinburgh in the middle of the night. I had never enjoyed running more, never felt more part of something, as though running itself were the destination.

Like an evangelical, I wanted to preach the benefits of My Way to everyone I knew. I would do this, I decided. I would no longer be the woman who encouraged those who already knew they wanted to run—I would convert them all! I would create a nation of runners, strong and proud! Then I fell asleep until the Wolverhampton train stop, my feet gently throbbing in my running shoes.

As the train pulled into Euston, I felt the excitement wear off. *It's understandable*, I told myself. *You were bound to feel a little high after an event like that. Just focus on the training for San Francisco—two months to go!*

Earlier in the year I had managed to secure a place at the Nike Women's Marathon in San Francisco, but in the whirlwind of other projects I'd undertaken, I had begun to focus more on the trip than the marathon. San Francisco had a certain hold over me, one that had only increased since my move to Brighton. And the idea of running in a women's marathon went directly to the part of me that had felt intimidated by the male bias at the other marathons I'd run.

But somehow, the idea of training for another marathon so soon seemed overwhelming. The excitement for running hills had blunted the reliable pleasure of endurance training. Excuses started to creep up like ivy around a solid house. I knew I could run a marathon, why stress myself out about this one? Was the point not proved now? I wanted to spend time with Louis before he was running himself. I wanted to see more of my London friends, feeling badly for not making it to parties on the nights before big races. I wanted my goals to stop shifting. Meanwhile, I was falling in love, and the disadvantages of hauling myself out of bed on a Sunday morning were no longer about tiredness but about leaving someone behind.

I plodded along the seafront in a daze. My running times slumped. Seams I never knew existed on my running clothes started to irritate. My hair would flap in my face, obscuring my vision until I was convinced I'd veer off the pier. My necklace tangled in the cord of my headphones. I was sure I was always running into the wind.

Perhaps, I found myself thinking, running was something I had done to fill a void. Maybe it was a pastime for the lonely, giving a shape and purpose to empty nights and weekends. It could have been a way to brag all along—a cunning disguise for elaborate attention-seeking. Now that all areas of my life were so much happier, it seemed like little more than indulgence, an unnecessary purgatory that I had inflicted on myself. What once held a certain nobility now seemed almost pathetic. If that were the case, perhaps I no longer needed it.

The thought solidified inside me, a crackling crust forming round my misgivings. A shiver ran through me. I shoved these doubts as far back in my mind as I could. I halfheartedly reassured myself that everyone felt a dip in enthusiasm from time to time, not only those in love. I continued to plod along the seafront, shaving one or two seconds off my time but little more. My determination to achieve a personal best in my next marathon seemed to be dragged further away with every passing tide. The idea of running after it seemed to be drifting even further.

"The only way to run a faster marathon is to get used to running faster," Adam told me as I huffed with indignation that my legs seemed to be refusing to run any faster. He assured me that the books were right—sprint training and shorter, faster distances were what I needed to focus on. I already knew I had the endurance. I hated sprint training; it was everything that had put me off running in the first place. The aggressive, leonine competitive instinct that required you to run *as fast as you possibly can,* turning your mind to nothing but speed and pain, repulsed me. The whole experience served only to remind me of those very first runs, when every single judder of my arse felt like my own body taunting me.

I could just about tolerate heading up and out of Brighton to the pretty Withdean athletics track, pretending I was Jessica Ennis or Steve Prefontaine as I attempted to hurtle across the terra-cotta tartan, which is the ridiculous name for the substance the track is made of. But when I was tasked with sprint training, I filled with purest despair. It is one thing to master the mental sleight of hand required to dress in tight Lycra and run in public, but to sprint up and down the seafront, thirty seconds or one hundred meters at a time, felt like tempting fate. I'm not built like a sprinter. I knew I looked like someone trying too hard, someone reaching beyond her capabilities. There was none of the pleasure of running and all of the pain. With every passing day, I felt like more of a fraud.

"What is it you are running from?" a friend asked when I said I wouldn't be able to make his Sunday lunch because I would be doing a half marathon.

"I don't know," I replied, flummoxed by the question. Was I running from something? It had never occurred to me that I was.

"You can't run from yourself, you know," he said with a wry smile.

I tried to focus on his paunch and the woolen sweater vest stretching across it. "Oh, I know," I said. "Me just keeps popping up at the finish line, wherever I run."

I laughed it off, but the question haunted me. A month previously, I had felt so proud of my strength and leanness; I now felt my own paunch mount a slight return, the result of lazy love-struck afternoons spent at the pub instead of haring along the seafront. I couldn't work out what I was running for, let alone what I was running from.

If I was happier now, doing work I adored and enjoying the love of those around me, was I merely some sort of traitor to all runners? Could such a thing exist? A fair-weather runner whose running is not dictated by the climate in the sky but by her own emotional climate?

Was it too late to pull out of San Francisco? My eyes drifted around my bedroom, looking for something to trip over. You can't argue with injury.

I kept these thoughts to myself for as long as I could. I posted the photographs of my Edinburgh experience online and lapped up the interest and enthusiasm from others. Yet it did little or nothing to reinvigorate me. I thought if I bottled it up, the feeling would pass, dissolve, sporelike, into the atmosphere. Bottling things up, I would learn, came about as naturally to me as sprinting.

One August weekend, I went to a friend's birthday dinner, a party I'd been looking forward to for weeks. I knew that my favorite people would be in attendance, along with bundles of good food and lots to drink. As I sat there and looked around the room, I realized it was exactly the sort of thing I hoped I'd be doing by the time I was in my mid-thirties. An enormous sense of contentment came over me, one with a dash of luminous smugness running. *This is it, I have achieved adulthood splendidly,* I thought.

There were about fifteen of us seated at makeshift tables composed of various people's garden furniture. It was the prettiest dining hall in Brighton, candles flickering and glasses of champagne being raised at regular intervals in a flurry of congratulations, celebrations, and happy birthdays. Two huge serving dishes of lobster macaroni and cheese were brought to the table, complete with elegant pink lobster claws. We gasped in excitement, and a dish was held in front of me. I reached for the serving spoon on the table and dolloped a huge rosy chunk on my plate, emboldened by booze.

"Why not? It's a party!" I said as I saw how much I had served myself. I hastily passed on the dish.

"I suppose when you run as much as you do, you can have as much as you want!" said a friend of a friend sitting opposite me.

"Well, exactly!" I said chirpily, vowing never to let on how little running I had been doing recently.

"How is it going, anyway?" asked another friend, her eyes twinkling with enthusiasm. I sensed a threat. This was someone who had previously asked for my advice on running in the past. I mumbled a noncommittal reply, hoping that my friend wouldn't notice. No one was listening; they were probably as bored as I was by the whole thing. She probably hadn't even stuck with the running.

"I'm sorry?" she said, clearly assuming she had not heard me on account of the general hubbub in the room.

Something inside snapped. I couldn't fake it anymore. I smacked the table, hitting it far harder than I had intended, causing cutlery to jangle and wineglasses to clink. Silence. Heads turned toward me.

"I'm just so bloody BORED of running!" I said, far too loudly for a now largely silent room. "I mean, what's the fucking POINT?" I raised my glass of champagne to my mouth defiantly. The secret was out.

"Oh, that's a shame," said my friend. "It used to make you so happy. You even got me into it!"

"Why, are you . . . not enjoying it?" another friend asked timidly.

I rolled my eyes dramatically. "I just can't see the point anymore," I declared. "I know I can run a marathon, I know I can get to Saltdean and back when it's raining, I know I beat a lot of people my age, and I know I will always be beaten by a lot of others. I don't need any of this. Why should I be trying sooo hard to get twenty minutes faster? What's the purpose? What would I ever do with that extra twenty minutes?" I waved an arm drunkenly. "I don't have to run far to find berries, I don't have to run fast to escape tigers. I just don't need to run. I can't work out why I ever bothered, really." I was on a roll now, unplugged. I seemed unable to stop.

Silence.

"I know, I know, it's awful," I added.

"It's not awful," ventured a voice. "It's just a bit of a shame. You were so passionate about it."

"I don't know why I have been trying so hard—I'm never going to win, so why am I so concerned about getting faster?"

"That never seemed to be why you were doing it. You always spoke about how happy it made you in other ways. It never seemed that much about speed."

I shrugged and scooped a second helping of lobster macaroni and cheese onto my plate, willing the focus to shift from me.

"Which marathon is it that you are training for now?" piped up a friend's husband.

"The Nike Women's Marathon."

"And where's that?" someone else chipped in.

"In San Francisco."

"Oh, wow! That is my favorite city in the world." Nearly the whole table was looking at me.

"Yes, I have wanted to go for years," I replied. "The race starts really early, so you see the sun rise over the Golden Gate Bridge. I've wanted to do it for a long time."

"That sounds fantastic!"

"What an experience!"

"It must be such an amazing way to see a city—they close all the roads for you, and people cheer you on, like visiting royalty!"

"Yes, yes, it is." My voice was smaller.

"If you can do that, why would you even bother about how fast you can do it?"

"I suppose I need a sense of . . . progression."

"So you see getting faster as the mark of progression rather than enjoying the experience more?"

"Well, yes, yes, I suppose I do."

When I woke up the next morning, groggy from booze and mildly ashamed by my churlish outburst, I wondered again why I had fallen out of love with running with such a thud. Was it the pressure of chasing times again? Did I think I didn't need it anymore? For the first time in months, I tried to solve a running dilemma the old-fashioned way: I e-mailed my dad. The subject header: "I just don't seem to be able to get any faster at running!"

His reply was succinct: "Why do you want to move fast when you are training for a marathon? Fast is relative."

When I explained my frustrations, how I felt I was running in treacle, how I wasn't sure I could be bothered, a similar reply came back: "It's not always about the time, it's about the experience, how you feel when you're out there."

He was right. Of course he was. I decided not to think about times, to abandon the ceaseless math project of working out paces and applying them to miles and kilometers. This in turn freed up some mental space for other thoughts while I was running, instead of endlessly checking my pace. Most crucially, it freed up space in my mind to try and enjoy the act of running once more.

For the final few weeks of training, I made a real effort to relax, to relish every step, to look forward to the process and not the destination. To feel my feet pushing the ground away from me, not feel my knees reaching forward. I got up one Sunday to run my locally organized 10K along the seafront and stunned myself by completing it four minutes faster and being in good enough shape to enjoy six oysters afterward with the man I had left sleeping ninety minutes earlier. Perhaps there was space for my love affair with running as well as other affairs of the heart after all.

Out of the blue, after years of following her career, I was given the chance to interview Paula Radcliffe at an event being held by her sponsor, Nike, on Clapham Common. I arrived huffing in the clammy summer heat. A crowd had already gathered to see her interviewed. As she walked out, I saw that she was with sprinter Carl Lewis. My heart was in my throat. The eight-year-old me who had been entranced by Lewis's prowess in the 1984 Olympics wondered what my dad would think of my seeing him in person.

The two of them were interviewed onstage, then Paula waded through crowds of fans asking her to sign things, to speak to them, to meet their babies. I was taken to the press area. As a result of my enthusiasm, I was granted interviews with both of the stars. I was warned that they would be brief, so I quickly prepared myself. I sat down to speak to Carl, a genuine icon.

He was glowing and I basked in his beam. His running shoes were box-fresh, and his running jacket was made of a silver reflective fabric. He shone in a way that only the very healthy or very rich do. He was immaculately polite and listened carefully to my questions. I asked how he would advise the woman who thought she might like to become a runner but had no idea how—the woman who believed there was a secret that needed unlocking. Who felt that she needed permission.

Mr. Lewis gave me a long, involved answer about how that woman should pick a route or a distance she wanted to run and then walk it every day for a month. He was convinced that this woman would then feel her "natural competitiveness" surge within and break into a run, desperate to move at speed. I nodded, smiling. I could kind of see his point, but inside me was a clear voice, one not wearing a silver jacket, that said: *I'm not sure any woman would see that through. She would have told herself she was wasting everyone's time halfway through week two. She would never make it to running.*

I thanked Mr. Lewis, choking back emotion as I explained how much it would mean to my dad that I'd spoken to him. Deep down I knew I wouldn't be passing on his advice. I held out for Paula. She would have the answer. Surely the most iconic long-distance runner of our time would provide me with the solid-gold nugget of advice that I could pass on to generations of would-be runners. I would be enthused anew. A nation of runners would be born! Inspire a generation!

Paula was unfailingly polite. Somehow I neglected to tell her about my recent and dramatic decline in enthusiasm; I pretended that all of my questions were for the novice runner. I asked her the same question—what would she recommend for that would-be runner?

There was a gentle pause before Paula answered softly, "Just go out and run. Just . . . go out and try it. That is the easiest way to get involved, to get hooked, and to experience what it can bring to your life. Do it. Go out and have fun, see if you like it."

"Yes, yes, of course," I mumbled politely. We chatted some more, and I thanked her profusely before heading for the tube, somewhat despondent.

Never meet your heroes was ringing in my ears as I boarded the train to Brighton. It had all been a bit of a waste of time. Neither of them had given me that fresh perspective on running that I had been searching for since Edinburgh. I began to wonder if it would ever happen. At home, I listlessly Googled a couple of the names Paula had mentioned in our chat: Ingrid Kristiansen, whom she had watched break the world record in 1985; trailblazing Norwegian runner Grete Waitz; and Joan Benoit Samuelson. I'd heard of Samuelson. She was the first woman to win the Olympic gold for the marathon.

It was only then that I learned that the marathon wasn't an Olympic event for women until 1984. I decided to find out more. Three hours later, I was still pinned to my laptop, slack-jawed at what I was discovering. There were these women, these incredible women, who had been fighting to run competitively for decades. As recently as the 1960s, they had been told that they couldn't, that they wouldn't, and that they mustn't. Women were forbidden to take part in public races, for fear of harming their femininity and reproductive health; some officials warned that distance running could cause the uterus to fall out. But some women just wouldn't be told.

There was Dr. Julia Chase-Brand, who in 1960 was denied entry to the Manchester Road Race in Connecticut. A year later, it was decreed by the body governing the race that she could take part, but her time would not be counted, and she could not run with the men. This did not deter her. She turned up on race day wearing a headband, a skirted running outfit, running shoes, and a necklace. The media was intrigued by her and followed her story with an uneasy mixture of support and patronizing headlines and questions, from "She Wants to Chase the Boys" to "Women don't run. You run. What are you?" They were flummoxed by her unapologetic combination of strength and femininity.

She was asked by an official to leave the race. She did not. And run she did. While the organizers had no intention of supporting her, the crowd—and other male runners—did. "The first guy I passed said, 'Go get 'em, girl,'" she recalled. She completed the race with a faster time than ten men—or that is what the records would show, if her result had been counted.

Five years later, Roberta "Bobbi" Gibb applied to run the Boston Marathon—deemed the ultimate marathon on account of it being the world's oldest and having very strict entry qualifications—only to receive a letter from Will Cloney, the race director, informing her that women were not physiologically capable of running twenty-six miles, and furthermore, under the rules that governed international sports, they were not allowed to run.

Bobbi's response? "All the more reason to run." The way she saw it, "I was running to change the way people think . . . If women could do this that was thought impossible, what else could women do? What else can people do that is thought impossible?" On race day, she was driven to the start line by her mum, wearing a blue sweatshirt with the hood pulled up and her brother's Bermuda shorts secured by string. She did a couple of warm-up miles, then hid in some bushes near the start line before beginning the race. Instead of jeering, the male runners were supportive, and she finished the race in three hours and twenty-one minutes. As she had been running without a place, the record books did not take note of her achievement, no matter how many newspapers did.

In 1967, Kathrine Switzer scoured the race entry form and rule book for the Boston events, only to discover that they were listed as "Men's Track and Field Events," "Women's Track and Field Events," and then a third category, "The Marathon," which specified nothing about gender. Although it was assumed that women were forbidden to run the race, the rule had not been expressly stated. Cloney, on writing to Roberta Gibb those years before, had not done his homework. Kathrine filled out the requisite paperwork and signed her name: K. V. Switzer, a childhood affectation inspired by writers J. D. Salinger and e.e. cummings. "Ever since I was twelve I signed all my papers K. V. Switzer, thinking I was totally cool." Then she got on with her training and prepared for the big day.

As the race began, Switzer had to lift her sweatshirt to show the race number on her vest, and as she did so, Will Cloney himself herded her through the starting gate without even noticing that she was a dreaded woman. Though she had made no attempt to hide her identity, the bulky clothes and terrible weather conditions had done it for her. As had happened with Bobbi Gibb, when the male runners realized who was in their midst, instead of reprimanding or reporting her, they cheered and congratulated her. "My hair was flying, I didn't try to disguise my gender at all. Heck, I was so proud of myself that I was wearing lipstick!"

Consequently, journalists took note and started to take pictures. They didn't stop there; they also started to heckle

Cloney's race codirector, Jock Semple, a man already known for his temper. Seething at the indignity of the race being "infiltrated," Semple leaped from the race truck and grabbed Switzer, screaming, "Get the hell out of my race and give me that race number." Classy. Switzer was understandably scared to death and tried to dodge him, but he had her by the shirt and was trying to grab her race number. "He was out of control. It was like being in a bad dream," she recalled.

Switzer's boyfriend, Tom—a fellow athlete and hammer thrower—was less afraid, and he body-blocked the race director, who "went flying through the air," leaving Switzer free to complete the race. Although her time was not officially recorded, she finished in four hours and twenty minutes. In 1972, in no small part due to the images of Switzer and Semple, the Boston Marathon relented, and women were allowed to compete officially.

It was even longer before women were allowed to compete in the marathon at the Olympic level. This barrier was left for Joan Benoit Samuelson to break. Having taken up running as rehabilitation following a ski accident, she found that "girls just didn't run in public. When I first started running, I was so embarrassed, I'd walk when cars passed me. I'd pretend I was looking at the flowers." Having run, and won, the Boston Marathon in 1979, she set her sights on the Olympics. By 1984, with considerable help from her sponsor, Nike, the inaugural women's Olympic marathon was set to take place. Only seventeen days before the Olympic trials, Samuelson suffered a knee injury and had to endure major surgery. To everyone's surprise, and in a triumph of fortitude, she managed to show up at the trials and win. Three months later, she ran—and won—the race in one of the most moving marathon finales of all time. She ran alone for the last few miles and entered the famous Los Angeles stadium to huge cheers, having not only completed the run of her life but opened doors to generations of female runners.

Her race wasn't just for the runners of the future. "I cried like a baby," said Julia Chase-Brand of the historic day. "She gave a tribute to all the women who made distance running possible. I took it as a very personal thank-you. Maybe she was me if I had been born ten years later."

By the end of my evening of reading and discovering, my mind was awash with images—how hard it is to run a marathon, let alone when you are not wanted, not counted, being spat at or physically assaulted on the course. These women weren't tedious gym bunnies or brainlessly competitive automatons. They had been rock stars of the road and gone on to become doctors and mathematicians. And there was I, a little cheesed off with the prospect of running a few times a week. A switch had been flicked.

The next morning I went for a run, chastened. My head was swimming with my discoveries. Those women weren't running to keep fit, to stay slim, or to impress anyone but themselves. They weren't chasing approval; they were chasing the effervescent joy of running. They were running to run, just as Paula Radcliffe had suggested. As I turned off the seafront and headed for home, I realized that she had been right. Sometimes, to find out if you are a runner, you have to go out and run. It turned out that I still was.

11

The Finish Line

*Only those who will risk going too far can possibly
find out how far one can go . . .*

—T. S. Eliot

L ondon gradually got smaller beneath us. Even though I
could see the city from the plane, it seemed very far away.
San Francisco seemed even farther. It had existed in my mind
for so long as a holy grail. The Golden Gate Bridge had transfixed me since childhood—it was one of those images you see
in picture books and cannot believe you might ever witness
yourself. When I was a teenager, watching films set there and
beginning to understand the city's unique political and cultural
history, San Francisco became the city of my dreams.

Running past the Golden Gate Bridge had been a big part of
the reason I wanted to run the Nike Women's Marathon, and I
was finally going to do it. I was so nervous at the thought that
I burst into tears and sat in a bit of a daze for the first hour of
the flight, scrolling through recent photographs of those most
beloved to me. I calmed myself down enough to sleep a while,

but when I got to the hotel and realized how alone I was, how far from everyone I knew and loved, I felt rigid with terror and utterly weak.

I closed the hotel room door behind me and burst into tears again. I was terrified. I opened my bag, got out my father's twenty-five-year-old woolen running top, and threw it on the bed, desperately hoping it might emit a bit of courage. Apparently not. I was going to have to find my own. I unpacked forlornly and looked at the contents of the cupboard. Two pairs of running shoes. A pair of tracksuit bottoms. Two pairs of running tights. Two running tops. And a dress. An unusual selection, when you looked at it laid out like that. But my friends had been telling me all year that it was unusual to spend so much time trying to get to the other side of the world simply to go for a run with a load of women you've never met. Nonetheless, I'd gone and done that.

I reached for my running shoes. I had arranged to go for a run with some other British runners I had gotten in touch with in the weeks before. We headed out from Union Square, where the marathon headquarters were, and down to the Embarcadero, the road running alongside the water. It was nine A.M., although my brain was convinced it was something else entirely. Both the water and the October sky were a perfect clear blue. My heart swelled as I caught sight of a bridge ahead of me, only to realize that it was not the right one. We continued along the water, past the farmers' market opening up, local artists setting up stalls, and boats delivering fish to the restaurants. I had made it! I was in San Francisco, where I had wanted to be for so long, and I had gotten there through running! My stride lengthened, and I felt the cramps and tightness from the flight dissolving away.

Later that morning I was invited to a press breakfast, where we were introduced to the athlete Allyson Felix. A superstar Olympian of 2012, she was one of the many magnificent women who had graced our TV screens over the summer, looking strong, proud, and goddess-like. To sit and chat with one of the women who had helped promote the idea that a useful body, a strong body, might be of more value than a decorative one, was amazing. Once again I was starstruck. I asked her about distance running, and she said she'd never run farther than four miles, and anyone who had was, as far as she was concerned, "someone with a great gift."

How had the simple act of putting one leg in front of the other made this possible? How was I living out the dreams of the little me on the sofa, legs dangling, unable to touch the carpet, watching the man soaring across the stadium in the jet pack at the 1984 Los Angeles Olympics? I felt more complete, more me, than I had in so long. Those weeks of despair during training seemed to melt away. I had a gift, I repeated to myself. I had a gift.

I wasn't feeling quite as gifted the next morning when my alarm went off at four-thirty A.M. I put on my running clothes, laid out as usual on the floor by the end of the bed. I rubbed Vaseline all over my feet, remembering the first time my father had told me to do so and how I had scoffed at him. I guzzled a cup of coffee and a carton of coconut water, my favorite pre- and post-run drink, full of electrolytes and far superior to those glucose drinks, in my opinion. I headed out through the lobby, where the concierge waved and wished me luck.

Union Square was swathed in darkness, but there was a buzz in the warm air. The huge palm trees were twinkling with fairy lights. The area had been taken over by the marathon, but now it was time for business. There were security fences going up around the closed roads, and several streets were lined with big yellow American school buses, ready to bring the runners home from the finish line.

I crossed the square and headed to an all-night diner where a group had arranged to meet. I had some toast and eggs, my usual marathon breakfast, while we took turns going to the bathroom and fixing our race numbers to our tops. Crowds were gathering, like a running zombie nation in the half-light. As ever, I found myself marveling at the myriad shapes and sizes of the runners. In among the crowd there were a few men, but all of them had marked themselves as either survivors of or those left bereft by the cancer whose charity the marathon was associated with.

Within half an hour, I had joined the throng lined up and ready to begin. I could just about see the stage, where my new heroine Joan Benoit Samuelson took the microphone and declared the start. I was going to be running in the same race as Samuelson. I was thrilled as the crowds inched forward slowly while daylight started to appear. Moments later, we set off.

We headed to the edge of the bay and ran toward the Golden Gate Bridge. The crowd fell largely silent, the thump of runners' feet the loudest sound around us. I could smell the fish and wondered how far they had all swum. I tried to remember the route map that I had studied so long back at home in Brighton and then on the plane. I had a pang of longing for home. Then I remembered the bridge. We were going to be there soon, weren't we?

Well, yes, we were, but so was something else. A fog the likes of which I'd never seen before. It was thick and claggy and coming straight off the water. I could feel the humidity settling in my lungs every time I breathed in. I looked around and saw how much visibility had been reduced. It looked as if there were only a few runners around me, not the hundreds I had set off with. Had it not been for the neon splashes on the odd running vest, I scarcely would have believed I was doing what I was. Fear crept back in. Would the whole run be like this? How would I know where I was going? The marks on the map that I had memorized were obsolete now that I could see no distance at all.

Then I noticed that we were running past the bridge—the Golden Gate of my dreams! All I could see of it were two concrete stumps looming above the water. It was early on in the race, and crushing dispiritedness was starting to consume me. How would I cope if the whole race were like this, so different from everything I had anticipated?

The delicate fabric holding my confidence together began to unravel. I wasn't sure if I'd make it without the visual and emotional treats I had bribed myself with. But then the landscape changed, distracting me altogether. A hill appeared, a huge hill. Five months of my breezy tweets in reply to anyone who had asked about the hills of San Francisco seemed rather facetious. I thought of my passion for hill running that summer, and I imagined that enthusiasm pushing me up the hill. And what a reward was waiting when I got there! There was a spectacular view across what of the bay was visible through the fog. No bridge, but as our heads bobbed up above the mist and clouds, I felt something approaching invincibility.

I gasped, not just breathlessness but excitement. The route was proving to be as astonishing as I had hoped. The views grew more and more spectacular as the mist cleared. I felt like an explorer venturing through the unknown and pushing myself to the limit.

As the halfway point approached, those running the half marathon started to peel away, turning toward their finish line, leaving the rest of us to do the final thirteen-mile loop. Though I wasn't even halfway done, a certain loneliness was creeping over me at seeing so many runners turn away. The distance I'd covered from Union Square felt endless, and the remaining distance seemed unfathomable. I longed for a running partner, a teammate, a companion of some sort.

Then came the texts. I had entirely forgotten, but Nike had created an app, which meant that my Facebook page could chart my progress with messages I had prepared in advance. When I crossed the mats at certain milestones, the chip on my shoe was activated, and Facebook loaded a message updating where I was. My heart surged as the messages started to appear.

"You are not alone, we are here with you."

"Hemmo! Run home soon!"

"KEEP GOING, DARLING!"

A photograph of Louis appeared, wagging his hands excitedly at the camera, wearing a snazzy pair of tracksuit bottoms. I wanted to hug my phone.

Next a simple row of kisses arrived. I was not alone. I never was and I never would be.

I waved goodbye to the half marathoners and looked around at the women who were left. It was unusual for me not to be surrounded by characters in costume or slower runners at this point in a marathon. This time the other women were just like me. They weren't freaks or hard-bodied obsessives or slaves to the track. They were women trying their hardest. Wearing photos of their family who inspired them. They were inspiring one another. We would run together.

We turned in to Golden Gate Park at mile eleven, and I

looked around at the natural beauty, stunned that I had made it here, that I was allowed to run this course. We passed waterfalls, unfamiliar tree types, and even a few buffalo in a field. After a few more loops, we came to the bay again. There were waves lapping on the beach at the side of the highway. The sea looked so infinite, so inspiring.

As the miles passed, I began to feel the ache of the distance I had run, and I started to feel drained by the effort. The flight, the homesickness, and the miles yet to come all seemed to be rushing at me. A wooziness came over me, and I gripped my phone tighter, willing some more messages to make their way to me. Again I felt far away from home and desperately lonely. But I kept going, one foot in front of the other, one foot in front of the other, keeping time with the waves. My energy was ebbing with the tide, and slowly, slowly, I felt myself lapse into a walk.

"No, darling, no!" said a voice to my right. I turned and saw a small, wiry woman, maybe twenty years older, smiling at me.

"Sorry," I mumbled.

"You don't walk, darling!"

"I don't think I can go on. I just feel so tired."

"No, darling, keep going, I'm with you." She had a strong South American accent. I asked her where she was from.

"El Salvador, darling, but I run all over the world."

"Wow, really? This is the first time I've run abroad. How many marathons have you done?"

"Fifty! All over the world! I love to run."

Her smile seemed as broad as the beach itself. Yet I felt horrendous. I thought perhaps I was going to be sick, as water started to course down the inside of my mouth in a way I had previously experienced only after a teenage night of too much cider.

"Come on, darling, it's less than two miles. We're going to do it. You and me. You are so special. What's your name?"

"Alexandra."

"Alexandra! Like Alexandra the Great! You are so special, keep going, keep going."

I was swallowing hard, trying to keep myself from being sick. I seemed to be seeing things in black and white as my vision blurred. Was this hitting the Wall? Wasn't that meant to be earlier in a race? Why was I ... so ... very ... tired?

My eyes opened with a start as I felt her grip my hand.

"We are nearly there, Alexandra! Look at the colors! Let's keep looking at the colors. Look at the yellow shorts. Can you see the bright yellow? Wonderful! Oooooh my! Look at her socks! Pink kneesocks, well I never! See the sky, Alexandra, see how blue the sky is now. Keep going, keep going."

And so she continued, holding my hand, coaxing me on like a child. I looked at the colors. I loved her. I wanted to be home.

"Look, Alexandra! We are nearly at the end! There will be firemen there. And necklaces. You are going to make it. You are so wonderful, such a special girl. Look at the colors, keep your legs steady, here we are."

I saw the balloons that marked the finish line, and I stared until I reached them, propelling myself forward with force of will alone. It seemed that someone had kicked me behind the knees. As the balloons grew closer, my relief was so intense that I could barely keep myself upright.

"Thank you so much thank you so much thank you so much," I sobbed, squeezing her hand. Finally, we crossed the line, holding hands above our heads. I collapsed into the arms of one of the tuxedo-clad firemen standing there and accepted the Tiffany's box he handed me on a silver platter. My marathon prize was not a medal this time but a necklace. I grabbed my friend and some of the others I had finished alongside, and I wept.

Sitting in the departure lounge at the airport the next day, I felt my phone ping, announcing an e-mail. I recognized the name in my in-box, but in my exhaustion, I couldn't quite place it: Kathrine Switzer. I opened the message, and only as I read it through the second time did I realize who it was from. Another of my marathon heroes, this time congratulating me on my marathon time. I had written to her months before to request an interview, and only now had she gotten the chance to reply. As a fellow runner, she knew how much it would mean to me to look up my time and congratulate me. My disappointment at a speed no faster than my Brighton marathon result turned to pride.

I felt a surge of new awareness: I was a runner for life. No matter what else was going on around me, no matter how long the gaps between my runs, no matter how high, how long, or how fast my races were, I was a runner. Once you have taught yourself that running isn't about breaking boundaries you thought you could never smash, and realized that it is about discovering those boundaries were never there in the first place, you can apply it to anything.

I sat in my seat on the plane, gazing out the window at the bay below, and put my hand up to touch my necklace medal. Was that the Golden Gate Bridge we were flying over? I stared, hoping, until we were above the ocean. I flicked through some notes and found a quote I had scribbled down. It was Julia Chase-Brand talking about her famous road race, the only woman among a sea of men: "Finishing that race was a defining moment for me. If I could handle that pressure, I realized I could go ahead and live my life as I wanted. I could do anything."

All of my races, my quiet solitary runs, my ridiculous rainy ones with friends, they all involved shifting a bit of blood around and getting my legs to take me from one place to the next. They had also been about so much more: the shame overcome, the courage discovered, and the exhilaration reached. Running had made my heart bigger, but only now did I understand in how many ways.

PART TWO

That was my story, and this part shall be about making it yours. Here are the answers to the queries I tormented myself with while I learned to run, as well as some extra ones I have been asked over the years. I was lucky to have my father for advice, but there were some questions he just couldn't deal with. I have been that woman typing "What happens when you run with big boobs?" into the search bar in the dead of night, and I have spent more hours than I care to count in running shops and at event expos, trying to work out what certain pieces of gear are for. Here is what I have found on my adventures.

Running style, fear of injury, and mystifying gear: It's all here. There is only one thing I could not find a solution to, and that is getting your period on the day of a big event. In running, as in life, sometimes it just happens—it's down to you to get on with it. Lots of tampons, lots of painkillers, and the certainty that those post-race carbs will taste even better are yours for the taking. Keep your head high and run like a girl.

12

Head over Heels

Listen to your body. Do not be a blind and deaf tenant.

—Dr. George Sheehan

Those who don't have the guts to admit that they don't fancy running often enjoy telling runners about the damage they're doing to their bodies.

Those who have a loved one who runs often worry about them being safe and well.

Those who run often let their imaginations run away with them when in pain.

Rumor and schoolgirlish whispers can create horrific anxieties about what is going on in your body when you are in pain. Sometimes you just want to be reassured that you are not being neurotic for seeking help about a physical sensation that is entirely natural. Sometimes you need to be told that you're not being idiotic for ignoring a potentially dangerous problem. It is difficult to tell what is a niggle or a natural development in your body and what is a real issue. Crippling pain can just as often be the result of panic, or simply needing a stretch, as it can be a lasting injury.

I spoke with Anna Barnsley, a physical therapist who has worked with runners and professional rugby players. She has also taught other physios and continues to run her own practice while following all of the latest research in her field. We did our best to get to the bottom of the top ten running myths. She is not only a hugely experienced physiotherapist and a fascinating coffee date but also a very patient woman who remained unfazed by my scrappy list of questions and medical vocabulary that wouldn't put a six-year-old to shame.

The single most important thing she taught me is that pain and your state of mind are intricately linked: Pain does not come from your tissues but from your brain. This does not mean that pain does not exist, because we have all felt it, but it is important to remember that it is produced in the mind. Anna explained that it's the brain's decision to create pain each and every time something painful occurs, and that decision is based on perceived threat. The threat can be compounded by all sorts of other stresses, creating the vicious cycle of leaving the house for a run in terror of feeling pain and thereby creating pain.

The Truth Behind the Top Ten Running Myths

1) Running will destroy your knees.

I don't run because I want to be able to bend over when I'm eighty.

Every runner has been told this by some smug twerp who doesn't have the balls to admit that he prefers watching the E! channel or playing *Grand Theft Auto*. These are both admirable pursuits, but don't pretend you chose them because of knee pain.

Each and every one of us will get wear and tear on our knees whatever we do in life. Some people will get more than others because of their individual biomechanics and some because of their lifestyles. We're all made differently, but we also use ourselves differently. Injuries will rarely be on account of one or the other; they will almost always be a combination of what we're born with and what we do with that. There will always be exceptions to this rule and those with serious injuries that rule out running. But running is not a hobby that ruins knees. In fact, it's often one that alerts us to more serious problems with our biomechanics and gives us the chance to deal with them before we're hobbling for good. For example, if I had never run, I never would have known about the problems I was carrying around in my pelvis, and I would have come a cropper later in life. I still dread to think what my pain level would have been had I gotten pregnant before the problem was rectified and I'd had something heavy to carry around in a pelvis that was in the wrong place. For the sensible recreational runner, there should be no significant problems. For a further look at knees, see the section on iliotibial band pain on page 166.

2) The high impact of running will give you a saggy face and a saggy behind.

Someone who runs a well-respected beauty salon asked me to find out if this is the case, as so many of her customers say they won't run because they dread getting a saggy face. Women regularly tell me statistics with great confidence: Running creates "twelve times normal gravity" on your face, as though the skin's elasticity is bouncing around like a pair of unsupported boobs. I don't know how this could be measured or what it means and neither did any doctor or expert I asked.

What I do know is that there is a level of what is called "oxidative stress" created through exercise. Oxidative stress is the production of free radicals in the body as a result of exercise, which can cause some damage to the skin's elastic fibers. But all of the other advantages that running provides—improving circulation, getting fresh air, reducing stress—boost your defense against free radicals, which easily counteracts that. The argument that oxidative stress ages runners is usually made by the kind of woman who tells you sternly, cigarette in hand, that you should eat only organic chicken, as factory-farmed is so full of chemicals. The single greatest threat to any runner's face or skin will always be sun damage. Sunscreen is the answer, not giving up running.

As for the saggy behind—it's bullshit. Running, especially up hills, is pretty much the best thing you can do to have a great bum. Even more so if you're supporting your training with some squats. People who tell you otherwise need to stop talking out of theirs.

3) Running will make you look like a man.

The debate about what is or isn't "ladylike" or "manly" is touchy and subjective. What one of us finds deliciously toned, another finds threateningly strong, and where some see femininity, others see weakness.

Assuming that people mean "very muscly" when they say "manly," rest assured that there is nothing specific to running that does this to you. Running is largely an endurance sport, which will build up your slow-twitch (or white) muscle fibers. Our muscles are composed of both slow- and fast-twitch muscle fibers: The former allow our muscles to take on energy on the move and convert it to motion; the fast-twitch (or red) fibers allow us to store power when we are at rest and put it into action in an instant.

Slow-twitch muscle fibers do not enlarge the muscles, as can be seen from the physique of Paula Radcliffe or Mo Farah. Fast-twitch muscle fibers do visibly enlarge the muscles, which is why a sprinter like Usain Bolt looks so much bulkier than a middle- or long-distance runner. Genetically, sprinters tend to be born with a larger number of fast-twitch muscle fibers, which is why those runners incline toward that discipline; likewise, long-distance runners in reverse.

Ideally, a recreational runner wants to develop both types of muscle fibers. Running hills and interval training are as essential to preparing for a marathon as completing the long runs. Interval training is the practice of repeatedly running shorter distances much faster than usual, with gaps for recovery in between. It is essential for improving cardiovascular fitness and breaking up the repetition of the long runs. The fartlek, which means "speed play" in Swedish, is interval training's more relaxed sibling, and it involves running fast bursts within the same run, rather than the more formal stop-start intervals. Integrating fartleks into your training routine will give you the instant power to accelerate through a low patch.

The bottom line is that taking up running won't turn you into Rocky. And even if it did, that would be your choice.

4) Running will make your boobs sag.

As discussed in the chapter on sports gear, running can indeed stretch the ligaments supporting your boobs, especially if you've got larger ones.

A bit of jiggling is okay and entirely normal. While a horribly restrictive, too small bra could affect your breathing, the swinging figure-of-eight motion made by a truly unharnessed pair of boobs is not ideal.

The solution is simple: If your boobs can't move around too much when you're running, they can't get stretched too much. There are amazing sports bras out there. Get involved.

5) Running makes your knees sound and feel like crisp packets.

It is a common sensation to hear or feel a slightly unnerving crunch or clicking noise in the knees on squatting or rising from a squat. This is called "crepitus." Despite sounding alarmingly close to "decrepit," it is not particularly dangerous. It usually originates from the patella-femoral joint, which is the interface between the kneecap and the trochlear groove of the femur, or thigh bone, which the kneecap glides along when you bend and straighten the knee.

If crepitus occurs without pain—which it does more often than not—then it is absolutely nothing to worry about. It is not something that will get worse over time, nor is it something specific to running.

However, if you are running a lot and it starts to become associated with pain, you should get it looked at. It could be your kneecap dragging on your femur and causing a bit of grinding, or it could mean that the cartilage at the back of the kneecap is wearing out. These are conditions that need to be treated by a professional.

The problem is often a biomechanical issue in which the kneecap is being dragged out to the side by structures on the outer thigh and lateral quadriceps—the latter can often become enlarged by exercise, which in turn causes rubbing that wears at the cartilage.

The noise does say "Danger!'" very loudly in one's brain, making it hard to ignore, but the situation is not usually as bad as it sounds.

6) Running's type of cardiovascular exercise is no good for weight loss.

The fat-burning zone that equipment in fancy gyms or swishy personal trainers refer to is any period of exercise when your heart is working at 60 to 70 percent of its maximum rate. This is probably what you feel like on a slow run, the sort of jog where you might admire the leaves on a tree or the bottom of someone running ahead of you. This pace indeed burns more fat than when you are exercising at a more intense rate. However, a slightly higher heart rate uses up far more calories, which is most important for weight loss.

So while there is some truth in the suggestion that running does not always work your body within the fat-burning zone, that does not mean it is no good for weight loss. Far from it.

7) Running makes you wee blood.

The kind of fuss I would make if I saw blood in my urine doesn't bear thinking about, so the fact that some long-distance runners see it as normal rather frightens me.

Seeing blood in your urine is not normal. It is not entirely uncommon in extreme athletes, but for the rest of us, it is indicative of a problem, not a nice blast of hard work.

If you pee blood after a long run, you need to make a doctor's appointment to check out your kidneys immediately. It is not known why blood is sometimes seen in urine after extreme exercise—the current thinking is that it might be to do with the way red blood cells break away during the exercise—but in an average runner, it is more likely to indicate kidney problems, dehydration, or overuse of painkillers, which are harsh on the stomach and kidneys.

Running does not do this to you as a matter of course, and it should never be ignored.

8) Running makes your wee smell of ammonia.

Running—or any extreme exercise—can make your wee smell of ammonia. But it shouldn't. If you get a whiff of that distinctive smell when you go to the bathroom, it means that you are carbohydrate-deficient and need to look at your diet. The smell is caused by the breakdown of muscle protein and is a result of running without enough of the right kind of fuel.

The brain needs glucose to function, and it cannot get glucose from fat, only from carbohydrates. While you may be a runner with body fat—you may even be a bit overweight and on a diet—the brain and body cannot access that glucose from your fat stores. Consequently, if you are attempting exercise without enough fuel, the body will start to break down proteins to access glucose. It is the amino acids in those proteins breaking down that causes the smell.

9) Running will cause vaginal prolapse.

I was shocked when someone asked me in all seriousness if this was true. I was even more shocked when physiotherapist Anna Barnsley did not dismiss the suggestion as entirely out of the question. Mercifully, running alone does not and cannot cause vaginal prolapse in a normal healthy person.

However, if you already have a tendency toward it, and childbirth is its most common cause, the high impact of pounding the pavement can bring it on. "But surely just a sneeze in the garden center on a sunny day could do that?" I asked Anna, who grudgingly agreed. She was, however, very firm that running also exercises your pelvic floor muscles, which counteracts the risk of prolapse by strengthening the area.

10) Running will make you die younger by using up your life's energy faster.

This suggestion divides the people I've mentioned it to into two neat halves: those who nod solemnly and say that, yes, it is entirely true and very worrying; and those who think I have finally become untethered from my already tenuous grip on reality for even researching the proposition.

It seems that this myth comes from the absurd idea that we each have a finite number of heartbeats in our lives, and by increasing your heart rate through running, you will use them up faster. There is so much research to show that life expectancy is extended by exercise that the notion is entirely absurd. Honestly, it is pure madness. Try to smile pityingly at the people who think it, as they probably also believe in witches.

Then there are actual injuries. Yes, sometimes running does hurt—and not just in the "oh my, that was a stiff wind this morning, my ears are stinging" sense. Here are the five most common injuries among runners, how to identify them, and how best to cope with them.

1) Iliotibial band (ITB) syndrome

By a significant margin, this is the most common source of pain for regular runners, particularly long-distance runners.

The iliotibial band is a fascia that runs down the length of the outer thigh from hip to knee. The repetitive action of running can put a large amount of stress on it, causing it to tighten and shorten after runs that are longer than half an hour or so. This in turn can cause fiery pain in both the outer side of the knee and up in the hip. It starts off as mild discomfort and ends up causing agony, leaving you in despair of ever running again and tackling staircases tearfully in reverse. It is a genuine torment for many runners, as it's impossible to tell whether it has gone until you have been running a while. It tends to make its reappearance when you're tired, possibly being rained on, a few miles from home, and feeling rather low. Like a bastard ex-boyfriend who sends you a flirty text every time you think you might be moving on.

While ITB pain is common, it is not insurmountable, and there is a lot that can be done to alleviate or prevent it. An excellent solution in the short term: Buy a foam roller (a large foam rolling pin–type object that looks not dissimilar to a buoyancy aid or a prop from *Gladiators*) and lie on your side massaging the fascia while you watch TV. While initially painful, this activity does a great job of relieving tension in the ITB and can be a huge help with the pain. However, it does not solve the problem of what is causing the pain.

In the long term, it is important to work out why the iliotibial band is shortening. There can be many reasons. The most common is because the gluteus medius muscle on the outer buttock is not strong enough or working hard enough. This muscle is the one you can see—the outer muscle lying on top of the others, or as I call it, "the Kardashian muscle." It is this one that turns the leg outward. In many of us, the leg may be inclined to turn inward, collapsing the arch and making the foot flatter, which is called "pronating." This lack of proper foot control as the foot hits the ground (which many fancy running shoes claim to eradicate entirely) lets the knees roll inward, creating tension on the ITB. This is generally a result of an underdeveloped gluteus medius and can be helped enormously by activating and strengthening the muscle.

You can investigate further, asking why your gluteus medius isn't strong enough. The answer will relate to the fact that instead of spending our days clambering over fields picking berries and chasing animals for dinner, we watch telly and wang around on the Internet. Bits of our bodies are unused like never before, so when we challenge them, our muscles are, quite reasonably, a little startled—at least at the outset.

While there are a lot of exercises online, as well as hundreds of "helpful" YouTube videos (which I suspect are more often watched by curious fourteen-year-old boys with a developing taste for physiotherapists in Lycra), it is always worth finding a professional who can look at exactly which muscles need to be reactivated and how. I am of the opinion that investing in a decent physical therapist and spending an hour working out specifics with them is a far better use of time and effort than trying on numerous pairs of running shoes and bleating to your loved ones about how your new hobby hurts. Doing a few (admittedly boring) exercises can generally do a much better job of solving the problem than spending hundreds of dollars on the right corrective running shoe or orthotic insert. Save your money for getting someone attractive to talk to you reassuringly while rubbing your thighs, and then buy a running top you feel a bit sexier in. Everyone's happier this way.

2) Plantar fasciitis

Plantar fasciitis sounds like a baddie from a science-fiction novel, but is in fact a sore foot. It is pain in the heel and sole of the foot that creates a realistic sensation of either running barefoot on hot coals or wearing through your heel altogether.

As with ITB pain, plantar fasciitis is most common when runners are at the peak of their training and taking on longer and harder runs. This is also when they can least cope with a painful and confusing injury. And as with ITB pain, it is caused by tightness in the body's fascia, in this instance, the foot area. The fascia is a tissue that each of us has covering the entire body. While I sat, gagging and squealing over my cappuccino like a first-time passenger on a roller coaster, Anna explained to me that the best way to imagine the fascia is to compare it to the film which you see when you pull the skin off a raw chicken: that opaque, slimy, cling-film-like connective tissue between the meat and the skin. For years I thought that my ITB was red and sinewy, like a piece of muscle, but apparently, I was living a lie.

The creepiest thing of all is that the fascia is one continuous tissue enveloping every single muscle and organ in your body. It wraps around your stomach, intestines, spinal cord, and brain. There is no beginning to it and no end, although it is thicker in some places, such as along the length of the thighs (the ITB) and under the arch of the foot. I find this simultaneously fascinating and repulsive, as if each of us has a never-ending sci fi beast within.

Medical science has only recently learned that the fascia has some bearing on communication within the body. We already know that the blood and the neural system play vital roles in transporting both messages and substances around the body; it seems the fascia can also communicate. What this means is that if you have tension in one part of your body, it will often create tension somewhere else. Hence the idea of "referred pain" and the popularity of reflexology.

Overstretching can cause inflammation of the fascia, and this is what is behind plantar fasciitis. Typically, it will occur in someone who pronates, as she will tend to repeatedly overstretch the fascia when the foot rolls over.

People mistakenly believe that yet more stretching will ease the pain. This will not help and may exacerbate the problem, particularly in the early stages. In the short term, get a bottle of water and pop it in the freezer, then use the frozen bottle to roll up and down the length of the foot like a rolling pin. That and rest will ease both the inflammation and pain. The injury responds well to rest, but in the long term, it is worth looking at your running style and the condition of the supporting muscles to the area.

3) Achilles tendonopathy

This condition once was referred to—and sometimes still is, in older reference books and the darker recesses of the Internet—as Achilles tendonitis, because it was believed that the condition was a result of inflammation. (The suffix "-itis" denotes inflammation.)

It was recently discovered that it is actually a physiological change in the tendon fibers at the back of the ankle, caused by repetitive overload on the area. When the Achilles tendon is overloaded (the diplomatic medical term for "overtrained" or "overused"), the body recognizes that it is under increased stress and starts to change its fiber composition. Over time a tendon that once had the springy qualities of a fresh stick of celery takes on the fibrous rigidity of a root of ginger: not so malleable and significantly stiffer. This causes the stiffness and pain that many runners are familiar with.

If you were to look at the tendons under a microscope, you'd be able to see that there are actually more cells, or a bigger "cellular matrix." This is caused by more blood vessels feeding in to it to try and make the tendon tough enough to cope with the overload. This becomes counterproductive, since to carry on running, you want a nice boingy tendon.

No matter how diplomatic the term "overload" is, Achilles tendonopathy is an injury caused by overwork. If the biomechanics of your body or the way you run are such that you put a lot of stress on that area, the most effective thing you can do is to rest. Think of it as an excuse to catch up on some box sets with your feet up. Running through the injury won't help, even if getting the blood flowing through the area makes it feel better in the short term.

4) Piriformis syndrome

The piriformis is a relatively tiny muscle that sits between the other gluteal muscles in the buttocks. One of the problems with the muscle is that it sits right over the sciatic nerve, so when someone is diagnosed with sciatica or back pain, she is sometimes suffering from an overactive piriformis muscle. This feels as if someone has jabbed a red-hot knitting needle into your bum from the side, as if planning to barbecue both your buttocks as a human kebab. It is also a hard location to describe when it is causing you pain. You're often reduced to pointing at your bum and gasping, "So . . . sore! In . . . there!"

There are so many surrounding muscles, tendons, and nerves that it seems impossible to articulate what you're feeling. For the greatest immediate relief, find an old tennis ball (spiky built-for-purpose rubber balls are also available in sports shops) and sit on it, rolling your buttocks around until you hit the spot. In the long term, the injury is usually caused by some kind of problem within the pelvis. As with iliotibial band pain, relieving the condition long enough to get through an event and working out the cause are two very different things. It's up to you how far you want to take it.

5) Ankle sprain

There is little that can be done to avoid this one beyond looking where you're going. It's easily done and incredibly common, especially if you're not concentrating. An ankle sprain is the result of placing your foot incorrectly and turning it over as you wobble off a pavement or out of a car, or by misjudging a piece of craggy ground if running in the countryside. The sprain refers to rolling the foot inward so that the underside of the foot turns in and the structures on the outer part of the ankle are massively overstretched.

I am particularly proud of having done this from a sitting position by getting up to go to the bathroom without realizing that my foot had gone numb. I took two steps on a waggling misplaced foot before the pain hit me, and I spent two weeks on crutches. Not strictly a running injury, but one that means I know this REALLY HURTS. Rest, ice, compression, and elevation (RICE) are your friends here. (these are what the RICE leaflets in doctors' waiting rooms refer to).

6) Stitch

Yes, I appreciate that I told you it was the top five injuries and a stitch isn't strictly an injury, but I am not sure there is any pain worse than a stitch. It paralyzes you with an evil pincer of pain and humiliation. Why does getting a stitch make you feel so idiotic? Surely you should have had some water or stretched properly, or done whatever it is that you're supposed to do to avoid getting one. Why does something so simple feel so utterly debilitating?

A small consolation is that no one really knows what you are meant to do to get over or avoid stitches; it turns out that there are all sorts of theories being expounded about what they are. The received wisdom is that it's a spasm of the diaphragm. The diaphragm is a muscle, so using it irregularly, or creating irregular breathing patterns by becoming out of breath at either the start or at a difficult part of a run, will make it contract out of sync and cause pain.

The best thing you can do is to try and breathe through it, to regulate your breathing by getting your rib cage to expand and contract. Beyond that, we're still waiting for the scientists' next big theory.

13

Getting Your Kicks

You have brains in your head. You have feet in your
shoes. You can steer yourself in any direction you
choose. You're on your own, and you know what you
know. And you are the guy who'll decide where to go.

—Dr. Seuss

*R*unning shoes are pretty much all you need to start running, and there are those who would argue that you
don't need them at all. You can get away with "these things I
used to wear in the gym five years ago" for a good few weeks.
But if you're running with a view to a specific event or you've
decided that you're going to go for it for a few months, a decent
pair of shoes will save you a fair amount of pain. The problem is
that you have to buy them. And buying your first pair of shoes
can be more painful than the harshest marathon.

Entering a running shop alone for the first time can be overwhelming. Attempting to buy my first pair of running shoes
was one of the most terrifying, humiliating, and dispiriting
experiences of my life, and I've interviewed Naomi Campbell.

All you are trying to do is find something that will take a milligram of the pain away from those first runs, but it can feel like an assessment of the most committed and intrusive kind. It should not be as hard as it often feels—after all, it's just buying some rubber and canvas to cover your feet. Since that first proper purchase before my first London Marathon, I've done it many times and in many different environments.

Top Ten Tips for Buying Running Shoes Without Having to Exchange Them for Your Dignity

1) Don't leave the shop with a pair of shoes that you find aesthetically distressing.

Running shoes are never going to be exquisite finery, but their strange stripes, swooshes, and signs can be peculiarly pleasing. Before I ran, I always found tennis shoes to have the most charm and had to be talked out of buying them on more than one occasion by those more knowledgeable than me. These days I care what my running shoes look like, but I am prepared to compromise for something that won't actively do me harm. Nevertheless, I remain convinced that the single most important thing about running shoes is that you're not repulsed by putting them on. If you don't want to wear them, you probably won't, and if you're not wearing them, you're not going to run.

2) Don't go shopping for running shoes in a short skirt with no tights.

Should you be actively seeking the attention of an eager

chap in shiny tracksuit bottoms, this is the ideal outfit: He'll be kneeling at your ankles for most of the process. If you just want to find shoes, perhaps wear something that'll make you feel a little less self-conscious while he's down there. It's best to plan ahead and wear pants or shorts or maybe something you might actually run in.

3) Allow yourself enough time.

It sounds so obvious, but as is true for many dreaded tasks, buying running shoes often ends up a result of a burst of "I'll just get it over and done with." The staff members measuring you often like to do their job properly, and this involves a lot of chat. Just go with it. Don't give yourself ten minutes and then succumb to the small trickle of sweat wending its way down your spine as you panic about how late you are going to be for lunch.

4) Set a budget before you go in.

Running shoes come in a huge variety of prices. There is no need to spend two hundred dollars on your first pair just to reassure yourself that your feet are not going to turn black and drop off. If you want fancy running shoes, go nuts—there are plenty around. But they won't make a big enough difference if you're just planning to get to the park and back for a few weeks. Summon the same courage required for walking through the department-store beauty counters while nonspecifically aged women with tangerine skin waft scent at you and talk lustfully of promotions. Eighty dollars is a reasonable expectation. You can pay less if you are smart about finding old models online.

5) Know what to expect.

There are three main methods that running shops use to measure what type of shoe you'll need. They will either film you running on a treadmill and look at the footage of what your feet and ankles are doing; ask you to run across a heat-sensitive pad that will show how your feet are landing when you hit the pad; or ask you to run up and down the street outside the shop while they watch. Clearly, option three is not ideal, especially if you are new to running. Running twenty yards in front of a shop assistant you've never met feels as natural as having a quick baby while you're asking the pharmacist where the shampoo aisle is. Increasingly, shops have more sophisticated ways of looking at your gait, and they are usually in fairly discreet areas of the shop. Doing some online research before you head out will help you key in on stores that bear discretion in mind.

6) Understand what the diagnosis is.

What the salesperson is looking to understand is which part of your foot hits the ground first as you run, how it hits the ground, and how a pair of shoes can balance that. The most common "flaw" is the previously mentioned and hugely bothersome pronation, when your feet roll in slightly as you hit the ground. There are running shoes that can offer support in your instep so that your knees and hips are not taking the hit every time you step out. Some retailers call this overpronating, some merely pronating. Some runners will underpronate, which is less common and sees your feet rolling slightly outward. If you do neither, you will be described as a neutral runner.

7) Remember that you are a work in progress.

This is hugely important. It is easy to cling to your diagnosis, having medicalized your problem, and to leave the shop with the most expensive remedial running shoes. But pronating isn't necessarily a permanent condition. Often it has nothing to do with the structure of your feet and is simply a result of a weak bum and thighs letting your legs flop in a bit. Take the expert's counsel into consideration, but don't let yourself be bamboozled. If the sales assistant winces and points at the most high-spec shoes in the shop, simply thank him for his time and spend the extra cash on an appointment with a physical therapist. Then go back to the shop when you *really* know how badly you pronate.

8) Know your pronating from your prolapsing.

When my sister decided to reignite her running career after Louis was born, I took her to Niketown to buy her running shoes as a birthday present. I sat unobtrusively, filled with a sisterly sense of respect and goodwill for her post-baby weight-loss mission, until I felt I needed to step in. That point came when I heard her confidently telling the assistant that she didn't pronate when she had her baby.

9) Leave your issues with the color pink at the door.

Pink is a pretty color. I am as devoted to my hot-pink NARS Schiap lipstick as I am to my rose-pink negligee. But pink skipping ropes and pink boxing gloves especially designed for "lady exercise" make me flush with an altogether ragey pink. However, where running shoes are concerned, you can drive yourself mad if you try to avoid pink.

It's the accent color of choice on a lot of running gear, and these days it's popping up on men's gear too. It's just a color.

10) Try to remember it's for fun. You're doing it for you.

14

Get Involved

Years ago, women sat in kitchens drinking coffee and discussing life. Today, they cover the same topics while they run.

—Joan Benoit Samuelson

*R*esearch has shown consistently that while health is the leading motivator in getting people to run, it is not typically what keeps them running. The social aspect does that. For many, joining a running club is a great way to find a community that provides motivation and may even improve your social life. For others, the thought of a running club is enough to bring on a more paralyzing attack of breathlessness than sprint training. As with finding the right hairdresser or the right husband, you often have to try a few first to find out what's right for you. Some are all about chasing time and competing against other clubs; others are about wider social movements, making running almost secondary.

Finding Your People

The Road Runners Club of America (www.rrca.org) offers an amazingly useful site that provides information on local running clubs in all fifty states, as well as guidance on finding the right club for you. Most running stores arrange weekly (or more frequent) runs. They are usually free, with proper guides and a coach at the back of the pack to make sure no one is left behind. They are a brilliant starting point and a surprisingly soft touch: I had feared relentless salesmanship but found only runners who wanted to find other runners, and trainers who could answer niggling questions about technique or guide your running for the rest of the week.

Many not-for-profit organizations offer expertise and cover race costs in exchange for your fund-raising efforts. The most notable organizations are the Leukemia & Lymphoma Society's Team in Training, the Arthritis Foundation's Joints in Motion, and the American Cancer Society's DetermiNation.

Mothers can visit seeMOMMYrun.com, a walking/running group for moms of all ages. Also, many races offer free group training runs to those who register. Visit the race website to see if they organize training runs.

15

The Perfect Running Style

*I'm a greater believer in luck, and I find the harder
I work the more I have of it.*

—Thomas Jefferson

There are entire books written about how to achieve the perfect running style. There is no perfect running style. There is a technical ideal, but those who have broken records or inspired millions are rarely the ones using it. The debate over what constitutes the perfect gait remains almost as controversial as the question of whether barefoot running is a fad or the right and natural way to run. It is impossible to dictate what is best for everyone, as our individual biomechanics are so different. I would no more presume to dictate how to run than to prescribe one specific dance style for womankind.

The single most important thing to remember is that we can all run. We instinctively knew how to run as children, and despite spending our adult lives in front of the computer or telly eating carbs, we are able to increase our stride in cases of emergency. There is no "I can't run." If you have functional legs and lungs, you can run.

However, those years sitting curled up on sofas or wedged into unsatisfactory train seats, as well as our own personalities and attendant neuroses, will have an effect on how we run when we go beyond fifty meters. To try and straighten these out from day one, or at least to give you the confidence that you're not doing yourself actual harm, you can follow some basic guidelines.

Running Guidelines for Everyone

Aim for a midfoot strike.

When I began running, I tried very, very hard to do two things in order to show as much willingness as possible: to bounce up and down springily and to reach out with my heels. I interpreted both actions as indicators of serious commitment to my sport and huge signifiers of great athleticism. I could not have been more wrong.

The ideal part of your foot to land on is not your heel. This is a myth perpetuated by cartoon runners, who spring into action with a fully flexed foot, and the huge aerated running shoes of the 1980s and 1990s. Barefoot runners believe that those big squashy shoes are responsible for making us all run incorrectly, and that we should be aiming for footfalls on our toes. In the absence of any conclusive research proving them correct, or indeed correct for modern, western runners, it seems the truth lies somewhere in between: We should aim to land in the middle of our foot—not right up on the balls of our toes but an inch or so lower, so we can give ourselves a bit of leverage as we leave the ground, without having to roll over the entire foot from heel to toe.

If we were to emulate the perfect running style, it would be the 1960s cartoon character Penelope Pitstop's. She has a lovely (if extreme) wide stride and lands correctly on her feet, even if she is wearing rather impractical white leather go-go boots.

I was wrong about the bounciness as well. It seems obvious, but it takes as much effort to springily trot along as it does to run with a more elongated stride, à la Pitstop. Aim for the latter, although perhaps not exactly like the latter. After all, we don't have Hanna-Barbera to sort us out in case of injury.

Never forget your arms.

You need your arms for running more than you might think. Try a spin to the end of your street and back with your hands shoved in your pockets, and you'll realize just how useful they are. Don't overthink it. When you're running, try to keep your shoulders down and let the natural momentum of your arms propel you. The best way to imagine them working is to think of the effort going into powering them backward, so that the swing forward is both relaxing and propelling. This feels counterintuitive at first, but once it clicks, it seems alarmingly obvious.

"Arms run hills" is one of my dad's favorite nuggets of advice, and reluctant though I was to admit it, he is right. This is where the arm swing is reversed as the gradient of the ground beneath you changes, and you need to push forward to help yourself up the hill. It feels as if you are punching the air and makes you thankful for those press-ups you've done.

Don't let yourself get too tense. Clenched fists with gripped thumbs or arms swinging wildly across your body, rather than loosely at your sides, will not help you. These actions will only transfer tension up to your neck and shoulders and leave you wondering how on earth a sport performed with your legs is making you want a neck massage.

Look after your head.

Heads are heavy—don't leave yours lolling around. It sounds daft, but if you spend twenty minutes running with your gaze directed at your toes, the weight of your head will drag you down and put a great deal of pressure on your neck. Of course you need to check where you're putting your feet from time to time, but try to keep looking up and forward so that your spine is straight and you can see a broader landscape.

Visualize yourself being pushed rather than reaching forward.

This too is something that I did incorrectly for months. Even after I got rid of my bizarre heel strike, I continued to reach forward with my knees, as if dragging my body behind them. You do have to run with your knees reaching forward, but it feels considerably easier when you imagine yourself being pushed from behind. Focus on your leg kicking up as you leave the ground, while your bum and the backs of your thighs are pushing you forward. This makes the biggest difference when you start to get tired and feel your body sagging. If you visualize a kindly (or perhaps just fanciable) chap giving you a shove from behind, you get a surprisingly large boost.

Do some complementary exercises.

No runner should just run. Part of achieving the perfect gait should also be about giving it a break. Should you get into running a few times a week, aiming to run a certain distance or in a certain time, you'll need to start doing a bit of work beyond your running to strengthen and support key muscles and guard against picking up any bad habits or mechanical imbalances that might ultimately cause you pain.

If you do some simple abdominal, arm, and butt exercises, you will reduce your risk of injury and feel significantly stronger. Pilates is also excellent for this. Go swimming, go for a long walk, or spend an evening in front of the television doing some stretching. It all counts.

Relax.

If you are terrified of running, your body will recognize that and produce adrenaline and tension. Try to relax and remember that you have chosen to do this. Warming up properly will help, as well as some key stretches afterward. You took time out of your day to enjoy your run, it won't last forever, and your body will thank you for it. Keep your shoulders down and your eyes up. Be proud of what you're doing: That is the most important element of any running style.

16

The Big One:

Everything You Wanted to Know About a Marathon but Were Too Afraid to Ask

> *"Man, this hurts, I can't take it anymore." The hurt part is an unavoidable reality, but whether or not you can stand any more is up to the runner himself. This pretty much sums up the most important aspect of marathon running.*

—Haruki Murakami

*F*or some, running around the neighborhood will provide more than enough stimulation. For others, me included, entering public events becomes a necessary motivation. Whether it's chasing an improved time or a medal, the thrill of the crowd's roar, or receiving the recognition of other runners, events can be worthwhile, whether you're entering a 5K fun run or trying to beat your marathon PR. Even though there is much to extol about races, they can really push your nerves. No matter how well you have prepared your mind and body, the tiniest of practicalities can trip you up. And even if they don't put a major dent in your race day, they can cause you sleepless nights. Here I offer you the benefit of my past mistakes and successes.

Doing It for Charity

Charity is the easiest way to take part in many marathons. Marathons or half marathons in big cities are hugely expensive to stage: Logistics include road closures, marshals, liaison with the police and emergency services, and the transportation and security of bags. While larger races usually have some random ballot places, the vast majority of spots are turned over to charities to allocate to runners who have applied for them. If you don't want the pressure of fund-raising for your first big race, smaller events are usually inexpensive to take part in, but be warned—what you lose in pressure to fund-raise, you lose in support en route. There is no doubt that I would not have got round my first marathon if not for my obligation to the charity. Without constantly reminding myself of the lives of those I was helping, I would have buckled under the weight of what I was attempting.

How does the system work? Charities buy places for a few hundred dollars each and give them to amateur runners on the condition that they raise significantly more money than the cost of a place. Every now and then a newspaper or a documentary will pop up discussing the "scandal" of how charities are expected to buy these places, as if they believed that every single person involved in manning roads, driving trucks, and checking bags could do it for free, but I rarely take much heed. A phenomenal amount of money is raised by people taking on a huge feat, and I struggle to see the problem with that. It is a truly humbling experience to share a race with those less able than you, those injured by war or disease, or those running in memory of loved ones.

What I do have a problem with is the small number of runners who take on a marathon in response to some existential crisis, commit little to the training over the six-month buildup, and then send out a handful of slightly passive-aggressive e-mails demanding a tenner the week before the big day. I believe that if you are asking people to sponsor you for a long-distance run, you have earned the right to ask, because you have taken on a daunting challenge. People don't sponsor you for the day you spend in a beautiful major city, being cheered and heralded by strangers as a hero; they sponsor you for the dark, lonely mornings when you get up before the heat has come on just to get that extra five miles done. They sponsor you for the parties you attend without touching a drop of alcohol because you have a long run planned for the next day. They sponsor you as a show of support to your loved ones, who are bored rigid of having you roll around on the floor complaining about your tight hamstrings. They sponsor you because you are paying tribute to others' pain by undergoing an experience that will at times hurt you.

During a period when you might already be busier than ever with running (and endless stretching), fund-raising can be an added stress. Here are some tips on how to get on top of the situation:

Choose your charity carefully.

Obviously, if your running is inspired by a specific person or event, this decision will be easier. Make sure you have looked into the charities offering places. It will make all of those wiseass "Why should I effectively be funding your hobby?" comments a lot easier to deal with if you know why you have chosen your charity. And it will make the darkest points of the run more bearable if you can properly visualize the pain that you are easing in others by experiencing your own.

Get a fund-raising page online.

The best known and most reliable is www.firstgiving.com. They have revolutionized the whole process; indeed, they have largely removed the horror of having to write down sponsors' offers and then chase the checks indefinitely after the event. They allow you to personalize your site with photos and text, to link to social networks, and to keep up to date with who is sponsoring you and when. You can either send individual thank-yous or one large group one after the event.

Be clear and honest about why you are doing the run.

If you simply want to prove to yourself that you can run the distance, be honest about that. There is little that people will spot faster than some spurious fear of brittle bone disease or a made-up uncle dying of an obscure illness. These tricks are entirely transparent, insulting to people's intelligence, and can do more harm than good. It's far easier to respect someone who tells the truth: "I have wanted to try running this distance for years, and as motivation, I have researched the charities and chosen to work with this one because of X and Y. I'm hoping this will help me get to the end, so do bung me a tenner if you have one going spare."

Use social media.

Don't use social media forty-eight hours before the event to post a jumbled selection of panicky messages in UPPER-CASE LOUD VOICE about how awful it's going to be because you've been so busy that you've hardly trained. No one cares, and they won't feel like ponying up their earnings if that's how you approach things.

Post regular updates on how the training is going—keep a diary on Facebook or hashtag posts and pictures on Instagram or Twitter. Let people in on what a struggle it has been on icy January runs, or let them whoop with you when you reach significant milestones. However lonely you might feel at times, no one runs these events alone, and knowing what you've been through is far more likely to inspire people to sponsor months' worth of commitment, not just one magical day.

Beware the power of the celebrity retweet.

Asking celebrities to post a link to your sponsorship Web page on their time line is of very little use. The vast majority of the time they won't do it, and when they do, their Twitter followers rarely click on the link. This is particularly acute in the week or so before a big event, when Twitter can start to seem like a jangly begging bowl being waved in everyone's face. It is significantly more effective—and appropriate—to ask specific people with whom you have a connection than to rely on the potential kindness of strangers.

Don't forget the power of the corporate cash pot.

Try asking your company for some corporate sponsorship. A lot of smaller companies are happy to put up a bit of money for you to run with their logo on your outfit, while others simply want to contribute to a healthy, worthwhile pursuit for their employees. If you work for a bigger company, it is worth getting them on board so you can send companywide e-mails promoting any events you hold to raise funds.

Be imaginative.

You don't have to ask people to sponsor you only for the race day. There is a world of other sponsorship ideas that you can dip into, from bake sales at the office to asking people for their unwanted things that you can sell on eBay to raise funds. Imagination is a more effective fund-raising tool than relentless nagging.

Be strategic.

Divide up the amount that you need to raise, or the amount that you are aiming to raise, and work out how many people you know who might be able to sponsor you a few dollars. Ask them. Then get creative with the others. Don't repeatedly ask people who won't be able to afford it; that's rude. It's easier to play to people's strengths, getting help from those with time and money from those with money.

Be polite.

No one is obliged to sponsor you. You have chosen to do this event. It is your responsibility. Don't be impatient if people don't immediately cough up. Be as lavish with your thanks as you are with your requests.

Maintain a sense of humor.

Running can be funny, undignified, and ridiculous. It's not necessary to be po-faced about threshold runs and lactic acid just because you are raising money for a worthy cause. Maintain a sense of humor—you might need it in other people before the end of your running adventure.

Work with others you're running with, not against them.

Find out if there are others in your area running for the same charity; if there are, try to coordinate with them. More than one set of contacts at a bake sale or a trivia night can make more of a splash and keep spirits high if you end up selling damp cupcakes at a drizzly fete with no one but the toothless guy from the booth next door for company.

Don't leave it until the last minute.

This really is one of the most important points. As with anything to do with money, avoiding the issue is not going to make it go away. If you feel awkward asking people, updating social media, or doing specific e-mails, you are still obliged to deliver the required money to the charity. The way they see it, your social anxieties are less of a problem than those being endured by the people on whose behalf they work.

Add the link to your fund-raising page to your e-mail signature or in the bio of your Twitter or Facebook profile, so you can alert people without having to address it directly. Don't ignore the fact that you've got a certain amount to raise. The charities will help you, but they can't do it all. As with the running itself, the only way to do it is to, well, do it.

Keep in touch with the charity.

Most of the charities that work with running events are very good at informing their runners where the funds are going and why they are needed. It is a tremendous motivation to visualize what the money can be turned into. There is usually a specific contact who can get back to you if you need help or have queries, and the charity always sends a team on the day to cheer you on. Make that connection if you can. Smaller charities in particular are hugely grateful for the funds, and the difference they make is immediate and tangible.

Looking Good for Marathon Day

The confidence that running has given me in my appearance is immeasurable. There are people who have seen me in my running clothes before or after a run whom I never would have let see me entirely without makeup five years ago. Public running events are occasions when there are professional and amateur photographers in abundance. I want to look good in those pictures. By "good," I mean strong, powerful, and inspiring. More than that, knowing that you don't quite look like death, even if you feel like it, is indisputably cheering.

Consequently, I have put an inordinate amount of time and effort into researching what beauty products look good, make me feel good, and, crucially, don't disintegrate before I have encountered my first glucose drink. These are my essentials:

Nail polish.

Nail polish is the perfect boost for running. I love it anyway, but when I am taking part in a public race, I have a positively Brontë-esque passion for sparkly flashes of color on my fingernails. I have run in Tom Ford Perfect Coral, Chanel Peridot (a greeny gold), and Illamasqua Rare. Before the San Francisco Marathon, I yearned for a certain sparkly topcoat that a friend ended up traveling across the whole of London for, as she knew how much a part of me my marathon nails are. It is almost impossible to chip or ruin nail polish while distance running, which makes it the King of Products for these purposes.

As far as my toes are concerned, I prefer to leave them bare, so I can survey any damage incurred when I get home. Make sure you cut and file your toenails about three or four days before the event so that they are neat but not so cropped that they leave flesh beyond the nail, which really hurts after three or four hours of running.

Eyeliner.

For my first marathon, I knew that I wanted to use one item of makeup that would stand out, stay the distance, and make me feel like a disco goddess even if drenched in sweat, rain, and humiliation. After much consideration, I went with an eyeliner that I'd used at my sister's eighties-themed hen party. Bright, almost violent green, it was MAC's Liquidlast in Aqualine, which takes about three days to remove. It didn't budge an inch on the hen night, despite our spending hours learning a dance routine and making a pop video to Whitney Houston's "I Wanna Dance with Somebody." I was finding neon sparkles on my pillow for days afterward, so I had absolute faith that the eyeliner would last a marathon. My faith was not misplaced. Despite at least an hour's downpour, I was still wearing it in all of the grinning finish-line photographs. Sure, it looked a little demented, but I was proud to cling to a little disco glitter despite the horrors of the day.

Eyelashes.

False eyelashes for running can feel very "Jane Fonda workout video," too close for comfort to brickish bronzer streaked high on cheekbones and slick lip gloss. But if your lashes are as translucent as mine, you can look like an albino rabbit in finishing photos, and mascara applied six hours earlier isn't going to make the distance. I'm not suggesting you apply falsies the morning of the race, which would be altogether too stressful, but I have become somewhat devoted to an occasional twirl with semi-permanent eyelashes done professionally in a salon. Applied individually to your own lashes, they make you wake up looking like Brigitte Bardot and are almost impossible to remove until they grow off with your own lashes. They are a firm marathon friend, and I save the requisite cash to make sure I can have a set on for big events.

Moisturizer.

Running does extraordinary things to one's skin. As someone who has always had very dry skin, I had anticipated that a few extra hours a week spent outside would leave it more parchment-like than ever. In fact, the opposite happens. The boost of circulating blood, as well as the sweat pumping out of my pores, gives me a glow that no product has been able to replicate. The salt of a good sweat is an incomparable exfoliant, as is the sea spray that blasts my face on seafront runs. That said, dry skin can be grim on long runs, and during the winter, I can feel rather battered. Clinique's Moisture Surge is my solution.

SPF.

As I've already touched upon earlier, despite the scaremongering about running making you look older, there is only one aspect to running that can age you: the sun. Hours spent under its glare in summer or winter can be terribly detrimental to the skin. I find it a little difficult to care too much about my skin aging given that, well, I am aging. But nor am I brimming with enthusiasm for a leathery face. Use an SPF moisturizer and a cap to keep the rays off your face.

A cap.

The ultimate runner's beauty accessory, it hides you from the sun and resolves the dilemma about what to do with your hair.

Hair ties.

A conundrum I have yet to solve fully. A ponytail can swish against the momentum you're trying to run with, a fringe can flap and fall in your eyes, short hair can become wild and unpredictable. Over the years I have relied on a selection of caps, clips, and bands to keep wisps of hair from making me murderous when I should be enjoying running with the wind behind me. Elasticated cloth hairbands ping straight off the back of my head and get lost in a bush. Buns unravel no matter how many pins I put in them. Having tried everything I can think of, I've concluded that the best things for keeping stray hair under wraps are old-fashioned plaits. I run almost Mormon-style. Yes, it's something of a girl-woman look once you're over twenty-five, but if your motives are entirely practical, as mine are, I reckon it's okay.

Packing for the Big Event

On the weekend of my first London Marathon, I was in a state of such high anxiety that I am amazed anyone was interested enough in my mission to turn up and support me. Perhaps my most neurotic behavior manifested itself in my preparations for the morning of the Big Day. I had become so terrified of forgetting something that for two whole weeks before, I had an immaculate display of everything I needed to take laid out over half of my living room floor. The trouble was, I kept having to use some of the things I'd need (my wallet, my running shoes, my house keys), so I had developed a complicated Post-it system in which different colors stood for what I was using. Looking back, I have often thought that I went entirely mad, but in hindsight my hypervigilance was not completely irrational. After all, I was about to leave my home and try to cross one of the world's largest capital cities with *none of my stuff*. Not even a little hobo knapsack. As I've already described, you can feel vulnerable handing over your bag before the race. It's gone, on a big truck, for hours. Your house keys, your ID, the lot. What I didn't know that first time is that the system that gets it back to you is awe-inspiring. On the day you register, you are typically given a large heavy-duty plastic bag with a huge number pinned to it. On marathon day, you have that same number pinned on you, so the chaps on the van can see you coming at the end, find your bag while you're being given your medal and goodie bag, and then present it to you as if by magic. "My bag!" I gasped that first time. "How did you . . . ?"

For what must have been the 2,343rd time that day, the volunteer pointed at the two corresponding numbers, patted my arm, and said, "Well done, you must be very tired." I was, but I was also happy to have my bag back.

Here's what you'll want to find in yours:

Warm, comfortable clothes.

When you finish a long run, your body starts to do some weird things, the likes of which I have experienced only during some of my most epic hangovers. You will be covered in sweat, probably looking as if you have just emerged from a shower even if you haven't made use of the cooling roadside showers. When you stop running, it's common to start shivering even if it isn't cold or raining. I enjoy selecting my most luxuriously baggy clothes to put on when I'm reunited with my bag. A nice wide-necked sweatshirt and some tracksuit bottoms with a stretchy rollover waistband are the dream. Peel off any of the sweat-soaked running clothes that you think dignity will permit (I'm always happy to stand around in a sports bra at this point; they're way bigger than bikini tops), then layer the baggy clothes over the remainder of your running clothes as soon as you can.

A pair of oversize socks/flip-flops.

The degree to which feet swell over the course of a marathon is truly extraordinary, and trying to put on any kind of shoe after you've removed your running shoes is like trying to stuff a baby back up the birth canal once it's crying in your arms. Huge socks that can be eased over throbbing feet are the order of the day, even if you have to walk on a bit of pavement in them. If the weather is warm, bring flip-flops.

Compression socks, worn to ease the ache caused by blood gathering in the lower legs after long runs, are significantly harder to get on. They can be stretched delicately over your throbbing calves and feet once you're home and showered.

Food that isn't too sweet.

After months of training, carb monitoring, and water slurping, you might feel that a huge bag of gummy worms will be exactly the treat for the end of your marathon. Think again. The toxic combination of sweating, breathing through your mouth, and eating and drinking sticky glucose products for hours will mean your teeth feel coated with sugar and your stomach is rumbling in revolt. At most races, they tend to give you sweets as they hand you your medal and T-shirt, so you're more likely to crave crackers, nuts, or chips, though chips aren't ideal for the whole "thousands of bags shoved on vans and lugged across town" bit.

Water isn't too important, as there is generally a lot of it about at the finish line of big events, but you might want to have a bottle in there just in case.

Toilet paper/wipes.

There will be so many places beyond the obvious that you'll want to wipe: your forehead, your feet, your sticky hands, under your arms, behind your ears. Basically, you will feel like a child who has just encountered his first ice cream sundae, and you will want to freshen up as much as possible until you reach a shower.

Painkillers/anti-inflammatories.

Even if you have no injuries and aren't expecting any, taking some ibuprofen immediately after a race can help your aching muscles and battered joints recover. Remember, medical staff at events will not give these to runners, as I learned to my cost. It's worth having some to share with others.

Tampons.

If you are a first-time marathoner, there is a strong chance that training will have confused your menstrual cycle a little. Be prepared for the unexpected. Whatever happens, tampons make useful cotton-woolly tools to mop up all sorts of other cuts and grazes that might be incurred en route.

Phone.

If you're not running with it, don't leave it at home. Though big-city marathons in particular can create a sort of "New Year's Eve 1999, everyone on earth is texting at the same moment" logjam, it is worth a shot in order to contact loved ones and find them at the end or let them know you have made it.

Wallet.

Even if you think you won't need any money because you've thought of everything you could possibly require, it's worth taking some cash or a card, so you can catch the cab home that you thought you would do without or buy the pint you were sure you wouldn't feel like.

Car keys.

As above. No one should put more effort into getting to a start line than in getting home from the finishing line.

Keys.

Don't lock yourself out. It would be the world's biggest known case of "FML" to be in eyeshot of your bath and bed yet unable to get into them.

Here's what you should have left the house with and discarded once used:

Baggy, disposable clothes.

At events, there can be up to an hour of standing around between checking your bag and crossing the starting line. At larger, less competitive marathons, there are often huge crowds and fancy-dress runners, and it can take well over half an hour for slower runners to get within sight of the starting line. If it's cold or raining, you're going to want to keep warm for this dawdling. It is beyond grim to start a race shivering, with muscles as tightly wound as your nerves. The best thing to do is either scrounge your brother's/boyfriend's/father's skankiest painting clothes or go to a charity shop and spend two or three dollars on a pair of baggy tracksuit bottoms and a hoodie that you don't mind throwing off, never to be seen again, once you're well under way and warm enough. It seems profligate, but most people do it, and the races are well prepared for it. Before the starting pistol has been fired, charity representatives are picking up the items by the side of the road and whisking them off to a better home.

Garbage bags.

While secondhand hoodies will keep you warm, they won't keep you dry. Garbage bags will. Yes, it sounds a little early Vivienne Westwood dressing the Slits, but it's an incomparably practical system. Just peel one off your roll under the sink, cut a gap in the bottom that's big enough to fit your head through, fold it up, and pop it in your bag. If there's a downpour while you're waiting, you can put it over your head. The bag will come down to about your knees and keep your running clothes dry. As you approach the starting line, you can slip it off and chuck it to the side. I tend to take a couple in case I see someone getting drenched; it would make a great if nerdy meet-cute. (This has yet to happen.)

Banana/sports bars/water.

You might not want or need any of these things, but they're useful to have, if only to share. By the time you reach the starting pens, breakfast can seem like a long time ago. Lunch will seem even further away. Nutritionally, I am not sure I have ever needed the snacks I've eaten just before setting off, but I always eat them in the spirit of not dying of sudden malnutrition.

Vaseline.

I tend to put a big scoop in an old makeup container that has been through the dishwasher. It's good to have on hand in case any straps or seams need relubricating, or to put on dry lips if it's a windy day. Again, it is considerate to take a bit extra in case someone else is in need. I pop it in a trash can before setting off.

A ballpoint pen.

I have forgotten to fill in the next-of-kin details on my running number more than once. I like to keep a crappy old ballpoint in my sports bag just in case. Make sure it's not anything inky that might run if it rains. It's easy to toss before setting off, as it's been especially selected for its nearly-at-the-end-of-lifeness anyway.

Your running number.

In the five years I have been running, the design of everything from water bottles to hair ties has improved almost beyond compare. Yet running numbers remain infuriatingly unchanged. How has no one tackled this? I despise them. They serve an invaluable purpose: They are your ID from the moment you surrender your bag until you retrieve it, and they carry contact and medical details in case of injury or security emergency. Yet given the slickness of almost everything else involved in public racing, they seem almost obnoxiously cumbersome. I often catch my wrists on the flapping fabric when I'm pumping my arms as I tackle a hill, and I have ruined a couple of tops by sweating through the fabric, which rubs against the number, causing the ink to bleed off the back. It is also impossible to affix the number properly if you have boobs. Men are fine; they just pin it onto their nice smooth man chests, popping it right above the stripe of their running club or sponsor vest. Women have to affix it over their stomach area, where things are flatter. This is also an area that you can't see if you have boobs, as well as an area you don't want to be blindly jabbing at with safety pins when you're already juddering with nerves. I've had to resort to asking women I've never met to help me out and am now resigned to pinning it to my top the night before, by lying on my back in my chosen running top like an anxious, carby ladybird, marking the spots where the pins need to go with a finger dipped in some water, taking off the top, and then pinning the number on while the wet dots are visible.

If men had boobs, there would be another way. Oh yes.

Safety pins.

For the mind-blowingly old-school method of affixing the aforementioned number to your running top. I hope with all my heart that one day they'll no longer be needed. I keep a small bag in my sports bag at all times.

Glucose.

These seem utterly disgusting and completely contradictory to all received ideas on health or weight loss. But running nine-minute miles for four hours uses over three thousand calories, and you'll need to replace them, fast. In the 1980s, my father used to eat chalky glucose pellets full of sweet orange flavoring, for extra energy. They were not unlike kids' chewable multivitamins you can find today. It was the greatest of treats for us kids to be allowed to have a corner of one; unadulterated glucose, it sent us into an immediate frenzy of hyperactivity. By the time I ran my first marathon, they'd been replaced by glucose gels—packets of pure glucose in a disgusting gloopy consistency. You have to rip off the top and suck out the grim contents as you run. Invariably, your tense fist will squeeze too tight, leaving you with a spurt of overspill that brings to mind an enthusiastic teenage boy and leaves your hand sticky for the rest of the run. These days I prefer to get my glucose in the form of jelly beans. Even traditional brands like Jelly Belly make sporty versions of their standard jelly beans. These are significantly simpler to ration than the jizzy gels, and easier to carry around. At some races they give them out, but not all. They provide an invaluable boost when all else seems lost.

Painkillers.

It is received medical wisdom that you shouldn't run with an injury or take painkillers in order to mask it. I absolutely agree with this advice. But I have learned the hard way that you can hurt yourself on the way round, or see someone else in pain, and a couple of ibuprofen tucked into a little pocket can make you feel invincible even if you don't end up using them. It is easy to feel as if you have lost your grip on reality while doing this, but cut the exact number that you need out of the blister pack and round them to leave nice smooth curving edges. A pointy corner that doesn't seem like a big deal on your bedroom counter can seem like a tiny satanic dagger once it's been jabbing into your hip through your pocket for three hours. The rest of the packet can go in the bag that will meet you at the finish line.

Phone/sports watch.

Not everyone likes to run with a phone, preferring to be reunited with it post-race. I use mine to monitor my pace and distance, particularly as the mathematics involved get exponentially more complicated, the farther I run. It's the flick of a thumb to check texts and tweets. I didn't realize how valuable it was until I ran the Brighton Half Marathon and one of the mile markers was in the wrong place. While I was trembling with rage as I saw my stats saying I'd run half a marathon while I was a few hundred meters from the finish line, revenge was sweet the next day when a huge proportion of runners complained en masse and the marathon organizers ended up amending everyone's times. This proved to me that, whether it's with a sports watch or an app, you should record your own stats in a public event, rather than relying on timing chips alone. If you don't want the distraction of a phone, you can switch it to airplane mode or simply run with a watch and/or heart rate monitor.

17

The Magical Secret

We run, not because we think it is doing us good, but because we enjoy it and cannot help ourselves . . . The more restricted our society and work become, the more necessary it will be to find some outlet for this craving for freedom. No one can say, "You must not run faster than this, or jump higher than that." The human spirit is indomitable.

—Sir Roger Bannister

That chapter title was a bit of a lie. Increasingly, I am approached by people who want to start running but haven't, as if there is a magic secret they're waiting to be told. There really isn't. As I've been told by every runner I admire, from Paula Radcliffe to my dad, the only secret is that there is none. You just have to start running. That said, here are the ten things I wish I had known when I started. As you'll see, much of it was advice from my father that took a little while to sink in.

1) Lacing up and leaving the house is the hardest moment of any run. You never regret it once you are en route. (Length of time ignored: one year.)

2) Nothing is ever as bad as your first run. No other run will induce that level of fear and pain. There are legions of people who believe that every run will feel like that first time. It never does.

3) Cover your feet in Vaseline each time you run for longer than about fifteen minutes. Not only will it stop blisters—especially if it rains—but it will mean deliciously moisturized feet on your return. (Length of time ignored: two years.)

4) Running in the rain is not perilous but, actually, quite good fun. It proves the adage about there being no such thing as the wrong weather, just the wrong clothing.

5) Don't eat too much before a run. Two bananas and a three-egg omelet are not necessary; that's just more to carry around with you. You are a healthy woman, not an elite athlete, so you have plenty of reserves. (Length of time ignored: three years.)

6) There is an extraordinary market in D-plus-cup sports bras that has clearly employed the skills of some of the world's finest engineers. If you rub Vaseline around your rib cage, you'll be even more comfortable.

7) Don't pay attention to anyone else once you're out there. They are either absorbed by what they are doing or looking on in admiration. If you can't do that, get a cap. (Length of time ignored: two and a half years.)

8) No one cares what you look like when you're running. Ever. Whether it's clean, cool, or baggy. Those first few runs *do* feel as if you're thundering down a catwalk surrounded by sneer-

ing professionals, but that feeling disappears as you realize you just want to be comfortable—and that the rare glance might not be so bad after all.

9) Stop stealing other people's running socks, they don't fit you properly! (Length of time ignored: five years and counting.)

10) You might enjoy it.

Acknowledgments

This book never would have existed if I had never crossed a finish line, so first and most heartfelt thanks must go to those who have been at my side as I did it, particularly my beloved Lottie Lambert, the magnificent Julia Raeside, Nick Brady, and Lila Frei. And of course Sarah Ballard, my immaculate "fragent," without whom I would have dared to neither run nor write, and with whom I am proud to cross the publication finish line.

The first steps of any book induce exhaustion, exhilaration, wobbly legs, and a terrifying sense that one's bowels could go at any time. So beginning a book *about* those feelings was particularly tricky. Early supporters were invaluable, with their unwavering belief that the book and the exploits it entailed were both possible and worthwhile. Thank you, Damian Barr, Clare Bennett, Grace Dent, Sophie Heawood, Melissa Marshall, Caitlin Moran, Jojo Moyes, David Nicholls, Rachel Roberts, Jessica Ruston, Polly Samson, Craig Taylor, and of course, my ever patient mother and her Olympic-level cheering skills.

Once the project was up and running, I reached its many finish lines only with the incomparable support of a rum collection of characters who were as consistent with their merciless teasing as they were with their steadfast pre-race cooking, midrace cheering, and post-race consoling skills. Thank you, Courtney Arumugam, Carol Biss, Joanna Ellis, Janey, Urmee Khan, Oli Lambert, Vanessa Langford, Jon Macqueen, Mike Moran, Joel Morris, Sarah Morgan, Kerry and Kieron Moyles, Geri O'Donohoe, Matthew Park, Jack Ruston, Julian Stockton, Jon Taylor, Eva Wiseman, and darling Louis, who provided such inspiration.

I am indebted to several people for their practical advice and for taking me seriously no matter how many childlike turns of phrase, ridiculous procrastination techniques, or ludicrous questions I employed. They are all masters of their professions and have been friends to me when I needed them. Thank you, Anna Barnsley, Kurt Hoyte at Run in Hove, Debs Hughes, Adam Kann, Josie Mitchell, Jay Stephenson-Clarke, Jo Taylor, Tim Weeks, and everyone at beautiful Café Coho in Brighton, where I both started and finished the book.

And thank you to everyone at Scribner and the Zoë Pagnamenta Agency, particularly Shannon Welch, John Glynn, and Zoë Pagnamenta for their consistent support of the book, my writing, and my determination not to have a pink book jacket—as well as their gentle but wise guidance through the U.S. publication process. It has meant an enormous amount.

About the Author

Alexandra Heminsley is a journalist, broadcaster, and ghostwriter. She is a regular critic on the BBC's *Radio 2 Arts Show* and appears frequently on UK television and radio. She is a contributing editor to *Elle UK,* and her work appears in the *Times,* the *Sunday Times,* the *Guardian,* the *Independent,* and the *Daily Mail,* as well as magazines such as *Grazia, Red, Top Sante,* and *Zest.* She was a judge for last year's Costa Novel of the Year award. She lives in Brighton.